I am food

Anthia has been working as a naturopath, herbalist and organic food, health and lifestyle educator since 1994, helping clients transition to brilliant health through the use of organic whole foods, medicinal herbs and spices. She runs Ovvio: The Organic Lifestyle Store and Naturopathic Clinic in Sydney's Paddington.

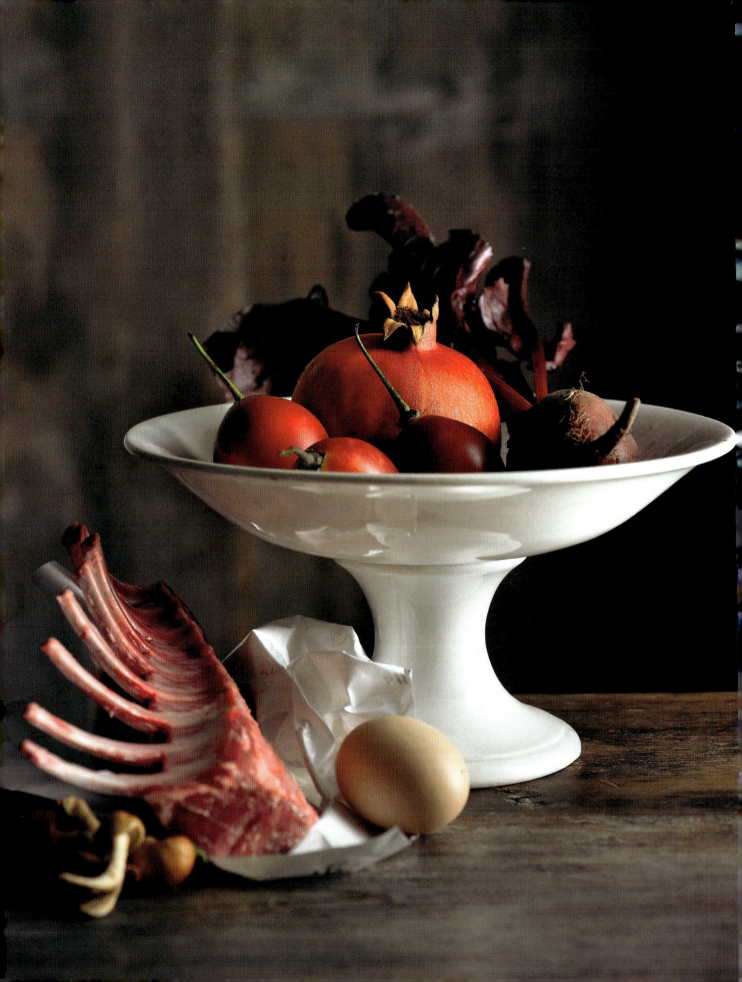

I am food

EATING YOUR WAY TO HEALTH

Anthia Koullouros

Photography by
Chris L. Jones and
Chris Chen

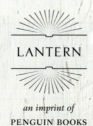

LANTERN

an imprint of
PENGUIN BOOKS

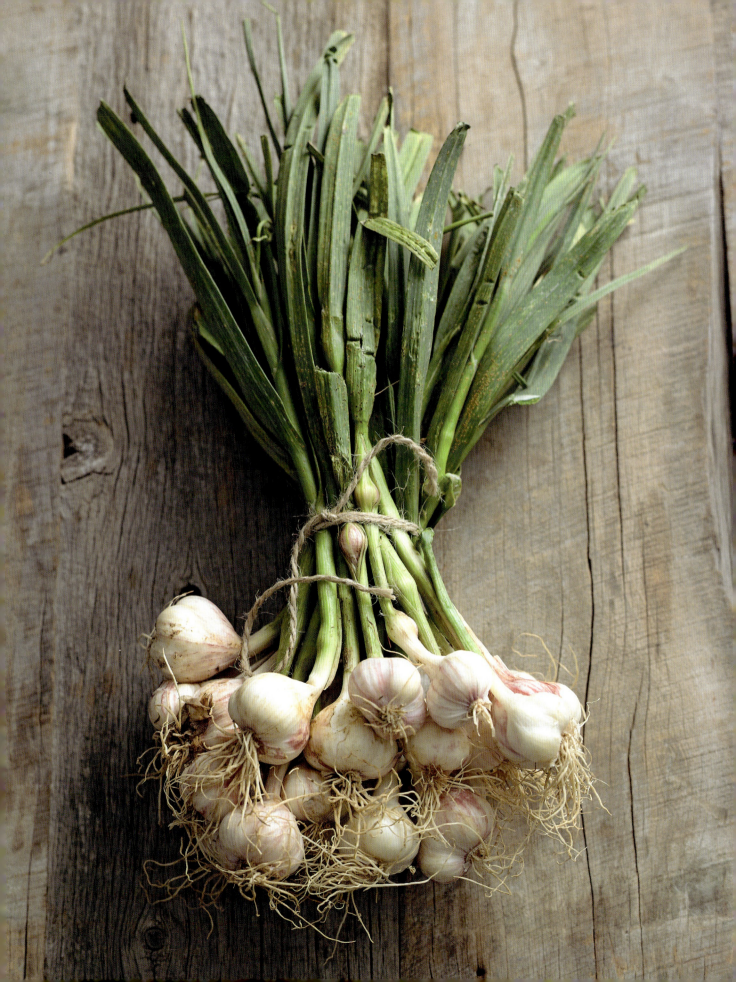

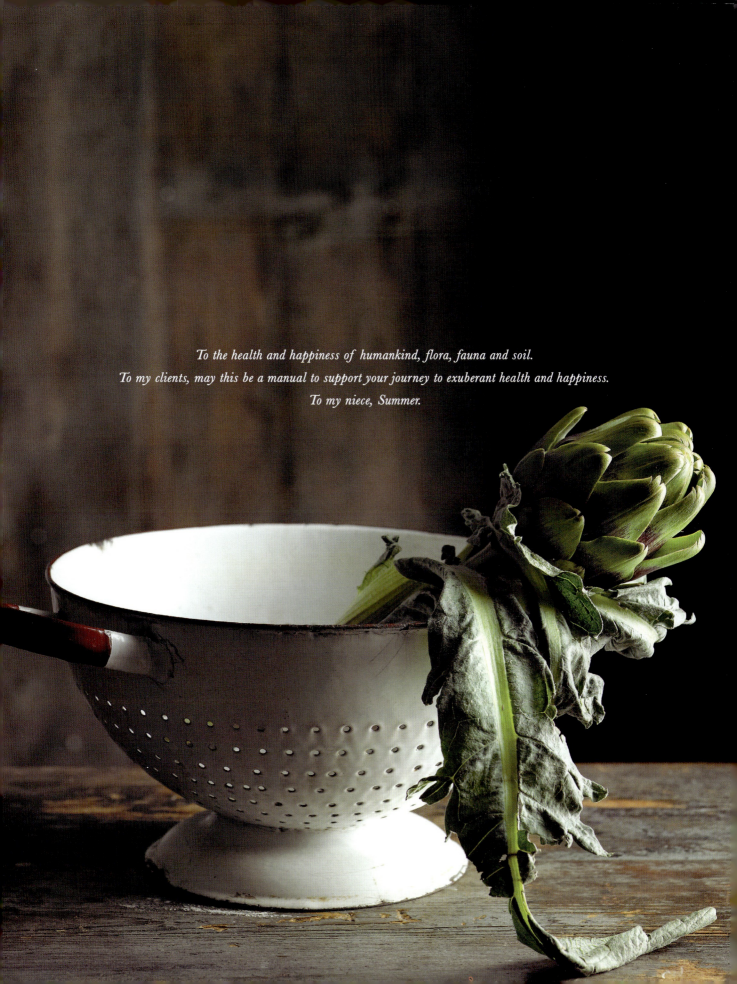

To the health and happiness of humankind, flora, fauna and soil.
To my clients, may this be a manual to support your journey to exuberant health and happiness.
To my niece, Summer.

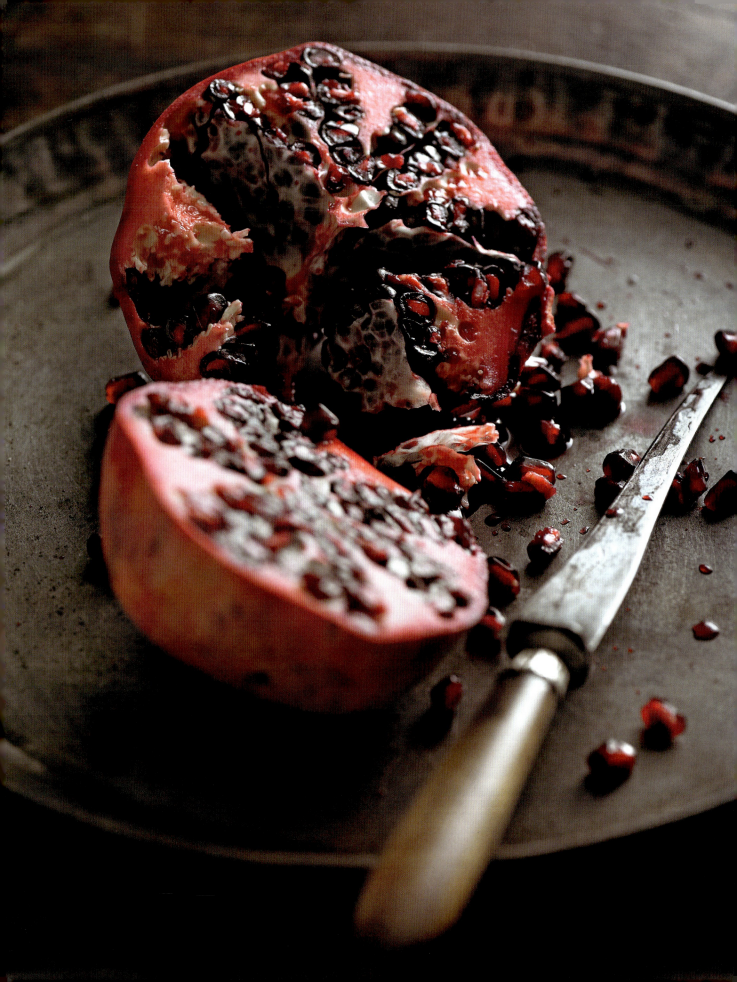

Contents

General principles – food for life	**1**
My top ten food philosophies	4
Modern diets and the way we should eat	7
Sourcing your food	11
Cooking your food	29
Choosing conscious, sustainable wholefood	37
Drinks	52
Cleansing – Making the transition	**55**
My wholefood shopping list	58
28-day menu plan	59
Herbal teas and food as medicine	65
Seasonal eating	66
Natural sources for vitamins and minerals	71
RECIPES	**77**
Breakfast	**79**
Light meals and sides	**95**
Dinner	**141**
Desserts	**183**
Basics	**211**
Resources	240
General index	242
Recipe index	244
Acknowledgements	247

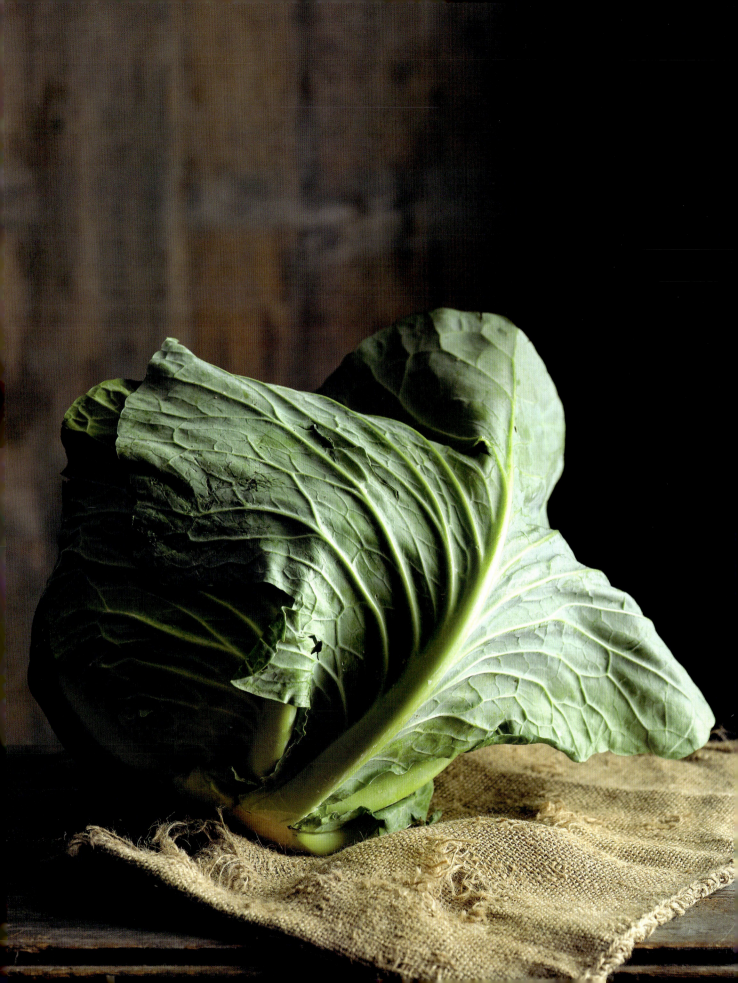

General principles – food for life

It is my passion to educate and inspire as many people as possible to choose products and take actions that add health, happiness, peace, love, beauty and truth to their lives and the lives of others. To achieve this I help people sort through their clutter and get clear about why they are feeling the way they are, and help them overcome the confusion that many people experience when it comes to health, lifestyle and nutrition. Education is the key, debunking myths and offering clear and simple, no-nonsense, fad-free, sustainable solutions to take care of their minds and bodies.

Every day I see clients to help them transition from a state of ill health to one of health and wellbeing. I also teach clients who are already in good health how to stay healthy. This is not only my job, but my calling, and I feel blessed to be able to share the gift of good health.

I believe health to be:
- Exuberant energy.
- Clarity of thought, and being able to create personal and health goals.
- Feeling balanced, grounded and alive.
- Being disease- and pain-free.
- Having no need for supplements or medications.

Two decades of naturopathic consulting have given me an abundance of knowledge, experience, wisdom and intuition that I wish to share with you. I believe the greatest tool I can give you is to teach you the ability to discern. I will encourage you to start thinking for yourself. I will toss the soil with you, shake up your beliefs and help you gain insight and clarity so that you can learn how to take care of yourself.

Many people make poor food and health choices and rely on shortcuts because they have limited time and it's convenient, because they don't know what's best, or simply because they feel overwhelmed and exhausted. Living on take-away and pre-prepared, processed and convenience foods is easy but in the long term these choices affect our health.

It should be a given that we have access to good, clean, healthy food for life. Yet it isn't. Malnutrition is actually prevalent in modern society even though we consume an abundance of food, fortified food and supplements. Many people have nutritional deficiencies and the reasons for this are manifold and often interrelated. See the 'Why Am I Nutritionally Deficient?' box, below right. Food, our very source of life, has been corrupted by money, power and a lack of education. There is also an enormous amount of confusing and conflicting information about what and how we should eat. We hear the words 'diet', 'low-fat', 'lean', 'enriched', 'processed', 'natural', 'organic', 'allergy-free' and 'superfood', all associated with food and health, and the barrage of information is overwhelming. Food manufacturing corporations, food marketers and diet dictocrats have the loudest voices, but the voices we need to hear are those of our bodies, our hearts, our intuition and the nature surrounding us. That's what I aim to do in this book: raise food consciousness. My message is, 'We eat what we are and we are what we eat.'

I am a champion of food that intuitively 'makes sense' – what your great-grandma would have cooked, pre-industrialisation, to sustain life and completely satisfy appetite and nutritional requirements. Food that funds farmers, not pharmaceutical companies, and is prepared according to traditional wisdom.

In a stressed-out modern society, it is even more necessary to obtain nutritionally dense food. Stress is insidious; it constantly draws on our health reserves, and – from years of clinical observation – I have seen that it underscores or contributes to many modern illnesses. In a healthy individual, acute stress, which can manifest as anxiety, irritation, panic attacks, lack of sleep, sensitivity, feeling overwhelmed, pain, fatigue, forgetfulness, anger or impatience, is speedily resolved.

It's when stress evolves into a long-standing, chronic condition that it becomes detrimental.

How does stress tax our bodies? I like to use the analogy of a bank account. We are each born with a unique nutrition and health 'savings account' – some are granted extra funds (via genetics, early diet, happiness, a healthy environment) while others enter the world already depleted. Each time we experience stress it draws on our reserves, siphoning credit away and gradually eating into our squirrelled stash. Eventually we enter the red – the timing is different for everyone, and once 'bankrupt', illness can emerge.

Why Am I Nutritionally Deficient?

There are many possible reasons for why you may be deficient in the vitamins and minerals you need. A nutritionally aware doctor or naturopath will consider the following questions with you:

Are you eating enough?

What is binding to your foods, for example phytates (see page 34), and preventing you from absorbing nutrients?

Are you eating poorly sourced food that has been produced via industrial farming practices?

Are you eating poorly prepared or highly processed foods?

Can you digest your food properly and absorb nutrients from it?

Do you have increased requirements resulting from stress, trauma or injury?

Are you exposed to heavy metals or other toxins which compete with or displace important minerals?

Are your genes affecting the way your body processes nutrients?

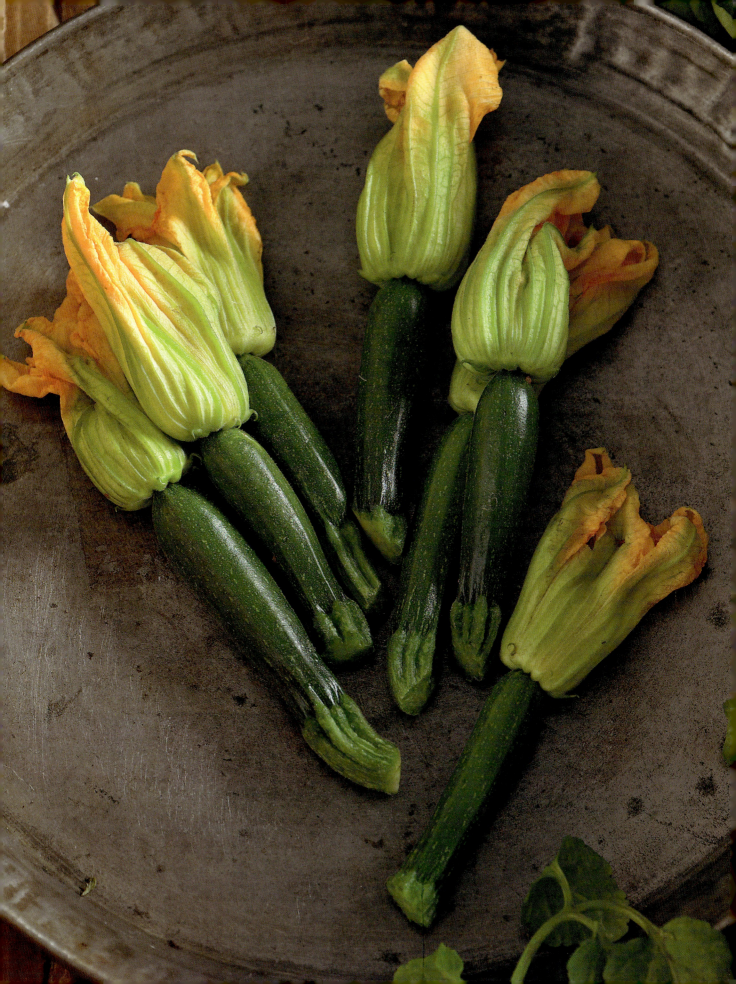

My top ten food philosophies

1. **Eat what we have evolved to eat.**
   Our anatomy and physiology dictate what we are able to digest and gain nourishment from. Modern hunter-gatherers, which is what we are, function best when we eat a diet rich in fresh wholefoods. These are fresh and cultured vegetables, whole fats and proteins from healthy pastured animals, non-farmed seafood, some well-prepared nuts and seeds, small amounts of seasonal low-sugar fruit and whole, unprocessed, cultured dairy products.

   Unfortunately many of us are addicted to carbohydrates, particularly wheat, rice, soy, corn and sugar because every convenient, ready-to-eat food is made of them. They are abundantly available to us because of mono-cropped industrialised farming and are often genetically modified. Carbohydrates are addictive because they are essentially sugar. We are also addicted to chemically processed vegetable oils and fats that are found in the same ready-to-eat foods. I recommend eating organically grown, low-starch vegetables as your main carbohydrate source and whole, unprocessed fats and oils sourced from healthy plants and grass-fed animals.

2. **Food is the foundation of health.**
   Food matters because we are what we eat. Food is nourishment and provides our bodies with the essential building blocks they need to heal and repair and keep us alive and functioning. That's why I called this book *I Am Food!*

3. **Eat what we can grow, raise, hunt and gather.**
   Healthy farming relies on rich, nutritious soil in which to grow our food: nurtured soil is full of life and nutrients. So let's buy our food from farmers who support this natural system, one that works with rather than against nature, to protect the health of our animals, plants, environment, seasons and climate. Eat seasonally, eat locally (to the best of your ability) but most importantly eat fresh, whole unprocessed food.

4. **Prepare food well by following our ancestral and cultural traditions.**
   The art of food preparation is often lost because we live in a fast-paced society which prefers convenience over quality. Preparing food well increases its nutritional density, and means it is more easily digested and assimilated. Choose to cook most food at 120°C or lower. Eat raw when suitable or soak, ferment, marinate or sprout your food to assist your digestion and help you absorb nutrients as well as possible. The recipes in the second half of this book will show you how.

5. **Cleanse, repair and support digestive function.**
   A cleanse is the bridge from eating industrially processed foods to eating whole foods to create a centred, clear, vital mind and body free from stress, pain, inflammation and disease. It detoxifies your body, repairs the health of your digestive system, restores immunity, balances hormones, eliminates chemicals in your environment, encourages you to get more sunlight and fresh air, and creates a healthy sleep/wake rhythm. Eating a wholefood diet after a lifetime of eating processed food may initially feel uncomfortable and you may need some herbal support. Weeding out bad gut flora and cultivating good gut flora is also important. Balancing your pH levels is done by toning your digestive juices. Digestive cleansing with each change in season will help this process.

6. **Observe and question your thoughts and beliefs around food.**
   What governs or inspires your food choices? Upbringing, food marketing, or spiritual or health concerns? Do you know what we have evolved to be able to eat? We are omnivores; we function best if we eat both plants and animals as our primary food source.

   Why do you eat? For sustenance and health, or for emotional reasons: distraction, boredom, anxiety, depression, indulgence, punishment or reward? Do you eat because you have to, or for comfort?

   How do you eat? With time, respect and gratitude? Or on the run, skipping meals or chewing food quickly without being truly conscious? How do you feel after a meal? Satiated, emotionally balanced and at ease, with a calm digestive system, or hungry, bloated, lethargic or uncomfortable? The way you feel is the way your digestion feels too!

7. **Experiment with different recipes and present your food beautifully.**
   But remember that however well prepared and presented, food is only as good as the ingredients it's made with, so begin with quality food from conscientious producers and sustainable sources.

8. **Beware of newly invented food categories.**
   The most insidious examples of these are babies' and kids' food, and snack foods. Aim for three square meals a day, rather than grazing on unsatisfying, processed Frankenfoods.

   I believe children are meant to eat what adults eat. Their first food should if possible be breast milk, followed by egg yolk, meat broths and vegetables from the age of four to six months, while still breastfeeding, until twelve months of age. If breastfeeding is not an option, create a natural food broth that resembles breast milk (see page 243 for where to find a recipe), rather than a processed infant or baby milk formula. At the age of twelve months a baby can eat healthy adult food. Simply puree it until they grow teeth. As children grow they can continue to eat what we eat. This will also save you time and energy as you will not need to cook separate meals.

   We are meant to eat whole foods: three square meals per day. We don't function well if we graze on snack foods made from unsatisfying processed ingredients.

9. **Be wary of government and institutional guidelines.**
   Unfortunately, conventional food recommendations are nutritionally empty and based on industrialised food production; they do not consider the source of food or the way it's processed. The current model has failed us. We still suffer from disease and ill health even though we follow institutional guidelines. So we try fad diets, supplements, medications and stimulants such as caffeine and recreational drugs to prop ourselves up. These are only temporary solutions; the body will eventually push us to have a forced rest, often through illness.

   Supplements are not a replacement for food and do not insure you against disease. In a society where we have an abundance of food, we still find ourselves deficient in common nutrients such as iron, vitamin D, zinc and magnesium, even though our food is often 'fortified'. The solution is to look at the source of our food and the way it's been processed.

10. **Learn to discern between real, honest food and food marketing.**
    Eschew packaged products, read labels and just eat the real thing! The packet or advertisement may say it is free of cholesterol, salt, sugar or gluten, or that it has been enriched with synthetic nutrients, but packaged food has been poorly sourced and highly processed. It has been altered. If processing has stripped something out and enriching or fortification adds something back, it isn't real food.

    Let's make it easy for ourselves and embrace simplicity! What food principles do you live by?

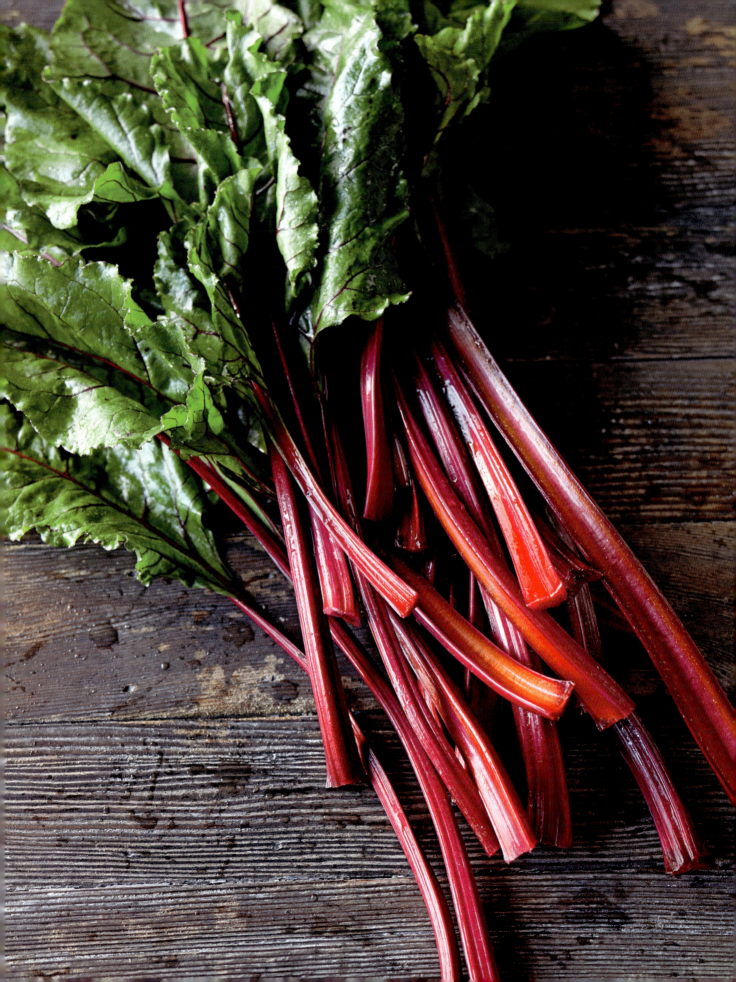

Modern diets and the way we should eat

The problems with modern diets are as follows:

1. They do not consider the source of food or the way it is processed.
2. Many doctors believe diet has very little positive impact on health and wellbeing.
3. If the connection between diet and health is recognised, a diet will often be prescribed merely to treat the symptoms of ill health, rather than addressing the problem at its root.
4. People believe the marketing peddled by giant food corporations.
5. Modern diets follow the government or institutional dietary outlines, which rely on industrial agriculture and chemicals to produce food.
6. Modern diets are often supplemented with medication and synthetic nutrients.
7. They include a great deal of processed and packaged, poorly sourced foods, fast foods, junk foods and 'ready-to-eat' meals, and are often 'fortified' and 'enriched'.

Health food diets

People who want to heal modern diseases often choose 'health' foods, but these are no different from ordinary processed foods: they are products and not real food. And people following a 'health food' diet often seek out many different health practitioners and try different diets, looking for a comprehensive solution to their health problems. Unfortunately they often remain unwell, ending up confused, overwhelmed and disheartened. Their diet works for a while, but the underlying issues are not resolved.

Obsessive diets or ideologies can be a mask for eating disorders. They often rely on supplements, 'superfoods' and 'cure-alls' in a bottle. They treat symptoms rather than addressing the real reasons for ill health.

Vegetarian or vegan diets

The common health belief behind these types of diets are that animal products are hard to digest, acidic and inflammatory. This is true if they are from unhealthy sources such as grain-fed animals. But what are your alternatives? For many vegetarians, they are industrially produced, highly processed, genetically modified, monocropped corn and soy products. It's important to think about the nutrients your body needs; meat, eggs and dairy products are rich in vitamins, minerals and fats that are essential to your body's functioning. We have not evolved anatomically or physiologically to be vegans or vegetarians. These diets often involve not only industrialised food products but synthetic supplements to make up for the nutritional deficiencies that result from not eating whole foods from both plant and animal sources. These supplements and industrialised foods support the production of chemicals as an alternative to real food. If you are vegetarian or vegan for ethical, spiritual, environmental or moral reasons it is important to take in the whole picture, and consider what is required to be healthy, without supplementation or medication, and free of disease.

Weight-loss diets

These are often low-fat, fat-loss diets, based on the premise that fat makes us fat. Processed, industrially produced fats do increase body fat. These fats, often in the form of polyunsaturated vegetable oils and fats, are high in omega 6 fatty acids, which are not good for you in large quantities.

They are found in meat from grain-fed animals, vegetable oils and vegetable fats found in packaged, processed foods, and in nuts, seeds, grains and beans (see Plant Fats and Nuts and Seeds on pages 42–3). They are called the 'fat bomb' and have pro-inflammatory effects in the body. A diet high in grains and legume carbohydrates, as well as starchy or high-sugar fruits and vegetables, will also make you put on weight. Weight-loss diets do not consider the source and processing of food and are often therefore devoid of nutrition. Weight-loss diets rely on calorie counting as well as meal 'replacements' and highly processed frozen meals to replace real food. Balancing reproductive, adrenal, appetite and metabolism hormones with liver cleansing through whole foods and herbs as medicine is the correct way to lose weight.

Cholesterol-lowering diets

These are often based on a fat-loss diet and a belief that cholesterol causes heart disease and death. In fact, our bodies make cholesterol naturally from carbohydrates, fats and proteins, because it is a vital component of the body's chemistry. Processed, industrially produced fats will clog our arteries and create inflammation of the arterial wall. This can lead to heart disease, as will unhealthy animal sources of cholesterol. A carbohydrate-rich diet has also been shown to contribute to heart disease. These diets do not consider the source and processing of food.

Acid/alkaline diet

Based on the premise that acid is unhealthy, these diets don't recognise that the pH of your body will balance out naturally when it is healthy. Your pH levels vary throughout your body; your stomach, for example, has strong acids to digest protein and control adverse microbial pathogens, whereas the small intestine is made alkaline by pancreatic and gall bladder juices. It creates this environment naturally, without the aid of alkaline supplements and fluids, to digest carbohydrates and fats.

Allergen-free diets

People are increasingly choosing allergen-free diets due to food allergies and intolerances. However, eating poorly sourced and highly processed food lacking in enzymes and nutrients, even if it is free of allergens, causes an unhealthy digestive and immune system and leads to intolerance or sensitivity.

Allergies and food intolerances are complex: sometimes they are genetic, but sometimes they can be brought on by our eating behaviours. Consuming a lot of any one type of food can create intolerances, as does eating foods we have not evolved to be able to eat.

An allergen-free diet does not address the underlying reason for the allergy, sensitivity or intolerance, even though eliminating allergenic foods can take the load off your digestive and immune systems. Choose healthy whole food substitutes. Be vigilant, as many substitutes are highly processed and contain synthetic ingredients which mimic the flavour, appearance, texture and nutritional content of the original food.

Be mindful that allergen-free foods are often just another marketing angle used by 'health' food companies to create brand-new products that yield high profits but little health benefit. Instead, always choose to eat whole fresh foods so you can keep repairing your digestive and immune systems.

Raw food diet

Raw food diets have some merit, especially when it comes to raw animal foods such as meat and dairy products. However, consider the source of the food and the methods you use to prepare it, as certain vegetables, grains, nuts, seeds and beans need to be prepared in ways that make them digestible, absorbable and free of antinutrients that bind to valuable vitamins and minerals and prevent your body from being able to use them.

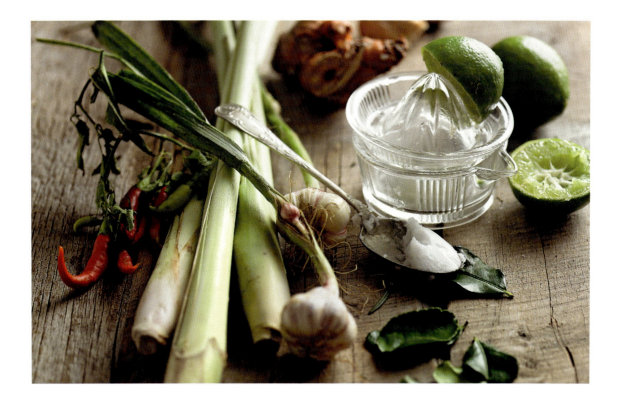

Juicing diets

These are a means to cleanse the body and lose fat. Vegetable juices are preferable to fruit juices, which are high in fructose and really no different from consuming sugar. Fruit juices produce the same highs and lows of energy, moods, appetite and weight as sugar.

Vegetable juices are better, with the pulp added back in and mixed with an animal fat such as some bone stock or melted butter. This helps certain nutrients such as beta-carotene transition to vitamin A. However, go carefully: certain vegetables, such as kale, broccoli, cabbage, brussels sprouts, spinach, chard, silverbeet and cauliflower should not be consumed raw and need to be cooked to aid digestion and eliminate anti-nutrients. If you have a functioning digestive system, it is better to eat food in its whole state than to drink juice, as nutrients are lost in the process. Your digestive system is a first-class juicer, extractor and blender.

For healthy juice ideas, refer to page 93.

The way we should eat

Taking a healthy, sensible approach to food involves some basic steps:

Consider the source and processing of food.

Consider the foods, recipes and preparation methods your ancestors and cultural group would have eaten and used.

Consider the holistic circle of life – the relationship between our health and wellbeing, and the health and wellbeing of animals, plants, soil and our environment.

Consider human anatomy and physiology and the evolution of human beings on our planet.

Develop a respect for food, understand the energy required to farm it and try to use it in a way that creates minimal wastage.

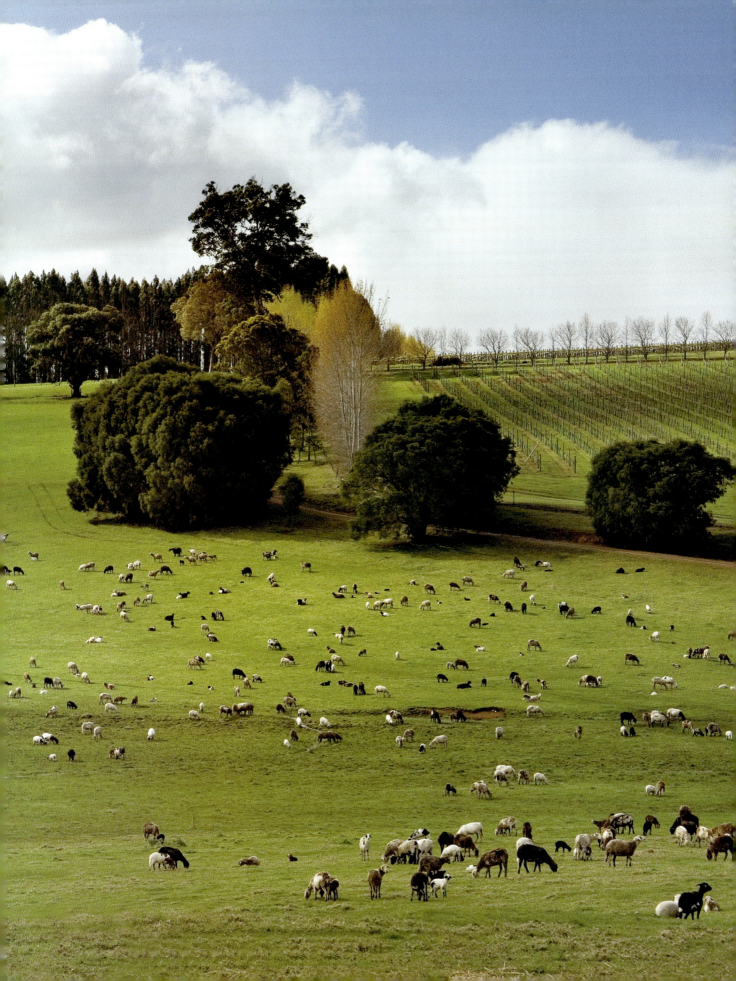

Sourcing your food

A food source is the origin of a food, drink or ingredient. The source and method of production will have an impact on the overall quality and nutritional value of that food. The quality and health of the soil that food is grown in is paramount in producing nutritious wholefood, as is being able to identify easily where the food came from. There are then the questions of how that food was treated or processed and whether it was marketed in a misleading way by food marketers.

TEN WAYS TO SOURCE GOOD FOOD

1. Eat seasonally.
2. Buy local produce.
3. Choose meat from pastured or grass-fed animals.
4. Buy open-range and free-range eggs and meat.
5. Buy from organic producers.
6. Support biodynamic practices.
7. Source from permaculture.
8. Choose GM-free produce.
9. Choose irradiation-free foods.
10. Buy chemical- and hormone-free.

Industrial agriculture

Industrial agriculture is the main source for modern food production. It has had a negative impact on the quality of food, soil and the environment, and therefore on people. When corporations take over food production, inevitably their focus is on making a profit, not on producing the highest quality, nutrient-rich food.

Long-term use of synthetic pesticides and fertiliser chemicals to achieve high plant yields has had devastating effects on ecosystems and food quality worldwide.

Corn, particularly, is the most over-produced and most subsidised grain in the US, a trend that is spreading to Australia. As a result, it is the most common ingredient found in every ready-to eat or processed food product. It is also fed to animals and found as sweeteners in other products we use, for example as sorbitol, a sweetener in toothpaste.

Monocultures

A monoculture is, as the name suggests, when a producer grows a single crop (usually soy, wheat, corn, rice, sugar or barley), often of genetically modified origin, year after year over a large area. The lack of biodiversity in this type of farming means that more pesticides and fertilisers have to be used, because the plant's natural resistance to diseases is reduced and the soil is depleted. Quantity overrides quality and the foods are robbed of their nutritive value.

Most convenience foods are made from these crops, usually grown, sometimes even organically, in a monoculture. They are highly addictive carbohydrates and we have become reliant upon them. But we have not evolved to be able to eat cereal grains, soy or carbohydrates as the main body of our diet. And quite apart from the effects on our health, industrial food production has environmental and social costs. Socially, the monopolisation of money and controlled distribution of food by large conglomerates means that smaller producers are unable to stay in business. The damage to our environment, from the soil to our climate, waterways and oceans, is irreparable, and the health of our animals is compromised when they are fed an unnatural diet to force an increase in production and yield. In turn, all these toxins and pollutants end up not only in our environment but also in our food and consequently our bodies.

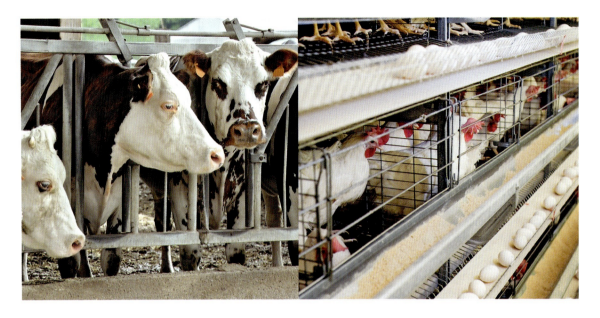

Factory farming

Factory farming means that animals have been jam-packed into confined spaces to produce a high yield of meat, milk and eggs at the lowest cost possible. The problem with this type of farming is that it requires antibiotics and pesticides to mitigate the spread of disease, which is exacerbated by these crowded living conditions. This produces unhappy and unhealthy animals whose meat does not offer us much nutrition. The meat of grass-fed animals, farmed as nature intended, contains much larger amounts of the vital nutrients omega 3, vitamin E and conjugated linoleic acid, compared to grain-fed animals in confinement.

Farmed salmon: the battery hens of the sea

Atlantic salmon is one of the most commonly eaten fish, and what we eat in Australia is mostly farmed. In fact, Atlantic (or Tasmanian) salmon is the most commonly farmed fish. This production method is cruel and they are often called the battery hens of the sea.

Salmon naturally feed on microalgae and small fish. Farmed salmon, on the other hand, are fed fish meal, wheat byproducts, soybean meal and feather meal (ground and dried poultry feathers). They are also fed carotenoids so that their flesh colour matches wild salmon. Because they are not eating their natural food they have very low levels of omega 3 (which you need) and the higher levels of omega 6 (which can be harmful) also found in grain-fed animals. Fifty per cent of world fish oil production is actually fed to farmed salmon to raise their levels of omega 3! Large numbers of fish are farmed or fished to feed farmed fish, fresh or in the form of meal and fish oil. This affects the development of the species and their natural habitat (large-scale fishing uses trawl gear and as a result of this there are a lot of wasteful discards or by-catch, including animals such as turtles that have been accidentally caught). Trawling also damages the bottom of the sea, affecting coral and seaweed life, which in turn damages the overall habitat and feed for fish and other aquatic creatures.

Fish oil, like many supplements, is not a complete food, and therefore cannot replace real fish, as the oil is extracted (usually with heat or solvents), purified and stabilised.

There is another problem with farmed fish, too. In the wild, diseases and parasites are normally at manageably low levels, and mostly kept in check by natural predators. This symbiotic relationship encourages species to live together in relative harmony. However, in crowded net pens salmon are susceptible to disease epidemics, and are thus fed large quantities of antibiotics, which end up in our bodies.

Sustainable fish and seafood
Each country has a Marine Conservation Society, which is a resource for choosing ethical and sustainable fish and seafood in order to protect our marine wildlife. They also offer information on seafood labelling and how seafood affects your health – a 'good for you, good for the environment' approach to choosing fish. Check your local society's website for details.

Get gardening!
Grow as much of your food as you can yourself. Gardening connects us to the soil, seasons, plants, animals, the circle of life and our food. It gives us a greater respect for food and where it comes from, stimulates our intuition, connects us with nature and its cycles, cultivates patience and most of all, it is an absolute joy to watch something grow that is so good for us. This is really the ultimate way to connect with and learn respect for where our food comes from. Choose heirloom seeds – traditional, open-pollinated, non-hybrid varieties that have not been chemically treated or genetically engineered. There are several companies operating in Australia that can send you seeds by mail order and I've included their information in the back.

Eat seasonally
Eating seasonally means paying attention to the times of year when a given type of food is at its peak and readily available to us. There are many advantages to buying and eating foods that are in season: lower cost, freshness, a natural abundance of nutrients and flavour, as well as a more natural growing or rearing method. Working with the seasons requires less human intervention, resulting in lower costs.

Eating seasonally allows us to better connect with the seasons as they occur naturally and supports our bodies to be more in tune with nature. Nourishing ourselves and our bodies with delicious, whole fresh food grown seasonally and ethically not only develops that connection but will keep us healthier, stronger and more resistant to illness and disease.

Eating seasonally creates periodic eating, which is the way our ancestors ate. Our supermarkets now represent all four seasons

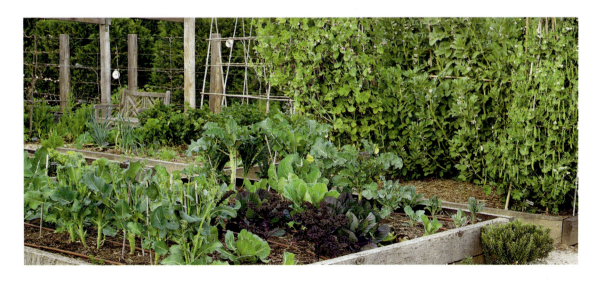

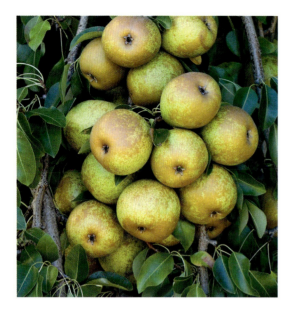

every day of the year because they buy food imported from many different countries, or that comes from plants or animals that are raised and grown industrially and artificially, no matter what the season is. But in our ancestors' day, food was very different. Winter was a time to 'hibernate' after autumn, the time of harvest, and in spring and summer animals grazed on pasture.

A change in season brings a change in weather and temperature, and this should dictate our food choices, cuisine and style of cooking. Eating salads and lightly cooked, cooling foods in spring and summer makes sense, as does warming up with soups, casseroles and slowly cooked foods in autumn and winter.

Changes in season influence our health and in some traditional cultures, certain foods were eaten based on their thermal qualities. These principles are the foundations of traditional Chinese medicine, Ayurvedic medicine and Hippocratic medicine. All ancient medical systems considered seasonal adjustments to the diet to be critical for good health as this ensured proper attunement of the body to the environment.

Eat local produce

Local food is food that has been grown or raised, produced, processed, distributed and eaten within one particular geographical region, close to the consumer. This not only has a positive effect on quality, cost, health and community but also enhances the economic, environmental and social health of that particular area. The bonus is that by supporting local farmers and food producers, the money you spend stays within your local economy, and fewer fossil fuels are used to get the food to you. Food grown and consumed locally is fresher, more nutrient-dense and better tasting, and helps support the sustainability of your local area and community.

'Locavore' is a term used to describe people who are committed to eating only food grown and produced within their community in order to build more self-reliant and sustaining food economies. Eating 100 per cent of your diet locally may be difficult to achieve as so many of us live in cities and more urban areas with limited or no access to freshly grown, locally produced foods. But now, with so many farmers' markets, locally grown produce is becoming more accessible to city folk, cutting out the middle person and connecting farmers directly to consumers. Look up your farmers' markets association to see what is grown in your local vicinity. You might not be able to get all your produce locally (coffee, some dried herbs and spices, and cocoa can be particularly difficult to find local sources for) but you might be surprised by the number of things you can find.

Choose pastured or grass-fed meat

Animals such as poultry, cattle, sheep, lamb and pigs grazed on vegetation are called pastured or grass-fed. These are animals raised as closely as possible to the way they would live in nature, allowed to forage in the outdoors with access to sunlight, fresh air, water and natural feed. This makes them healthier and they therefore require less

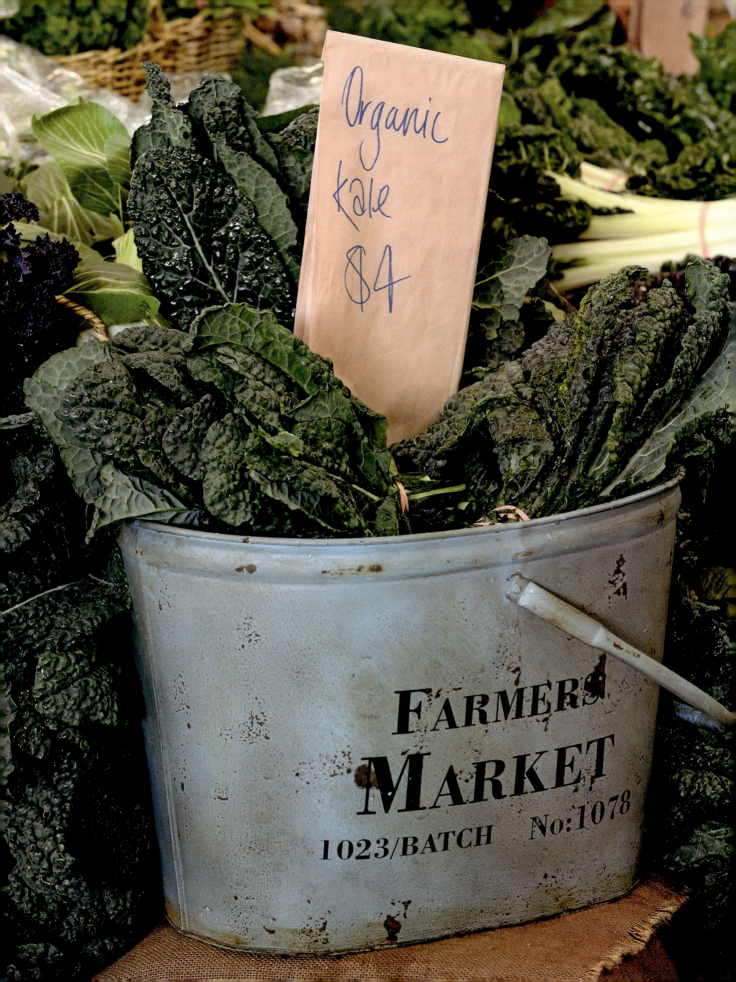

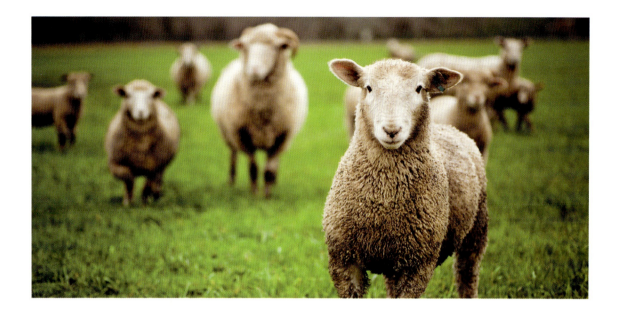

medical intervention, antibiotics and vaccines. Grass-fed is good for us, the animals, the environment and farmers.

Be sceptical, though. The words 'grass fed' can also be used to sell animals that are partially grass fed. Ask your retailer or butcher whether the animals have been grass fed their entire lives. It is common practice to finish animals in feedlots in the last 120 days of their life. This fattens them up quickly and produces a greater carcass weight, but it contributes to poor health and the quality of the meat is compromised. The animals have more body fat and less healthy lean muscle tissue, which is what you really want.

And be aware, also, that organic doesn't always mean grass-fed. Animals may be kept in confined spaces and fed on organic grain feed. This is no different from a human eating organic processed products rather than organic fresh whole foods.

Choose open-range and free-range eggs

Free-range animals are those that have some access to the outdoors. How much access, how often, and how big the outdoor area is can vary greatly and the term 'free range' may be used differently depending on the country and its laws.

'Cage-free' eggs are also known as 'barn-laid' eggs and can actually be called free-range eggs. Hens aren't kept in cages but instead are free to roam in large sheds.

'Open range' eggs means chooks roaming outside on pasture, protected by dogs from predators and coming in to roost at night in a sheltered chicken house. Hens, whether they are organic, open-range, cage-free or free-range, are supplemented with feed. The best way to choose eggs is to learn more about the farm. The healthiest, most ethical choice is open range supplemented with organic, natural feed that is free of genetically modified ingredients.

Eat organically grown foods

Organic farming basically means growing food without using chemical fertilisers or pesticides. Pay close attention to what you're buying, though. Known as 'industrial organics', organic food production can still follow the same unnatural methods of farming as industrial agriculture. Food is often grown out of season and travels long distances, and may also be exported. Buying certified organic or biodynamic whole fruit and vegetables that

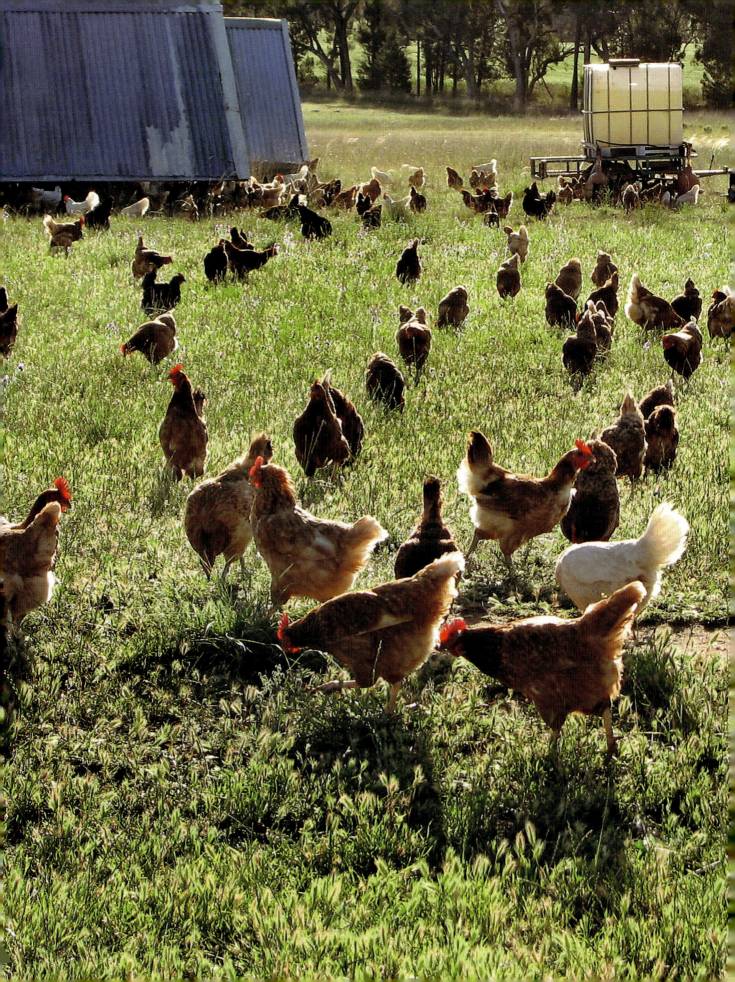

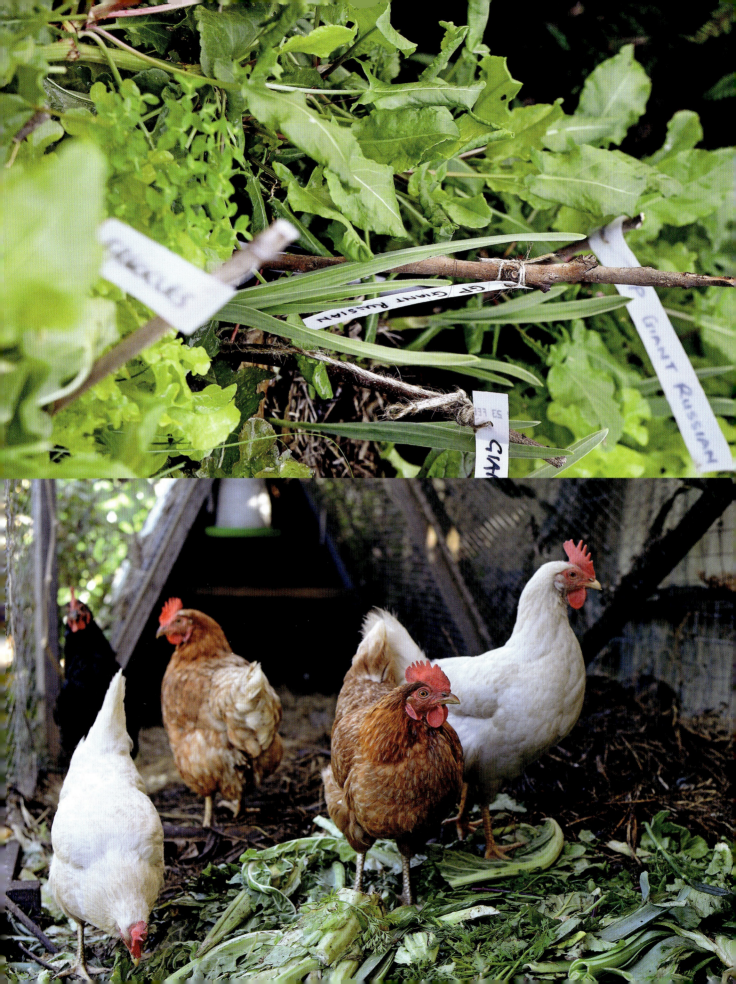

are grown locally or regionally is really the best option when sourcing quality produce. They will be seasonally and ethically grown in accordance with organic certification guidelines. If you choose to buy produce that is locally grown and chemical-free, but not necessarily certified organic, visit the farm or speak to the farmer; then you can ask questions and get assurance that the produce is being grown without chemical intervention. There are several bodies with differing standards for what's considered organic in Australia; I have given a reference to a website where these are listed with explanations on page 243.

Seasonal, locally grown, organic whole fruit and vegetables are the best current option for sourcing quality produce. Pastured animals are better than animals simply described as 'organic', unless they are both organic and pastured. Organic processed and packaged foods are no better than conventional packaged foods because even though the source might be good, the processing methods destroy the natural nutrients. Only choose packaged foods which have simple ingredients such as raw coconut oil or dried herbs and spices.

Biodynamic farming is all about improving soil quality and reversing soil degradation. A soil rich in humus and biological activity is a prerequisite for any sustainable agricultural system. Biodynamic practices do not rely on artificial fertilisers, though some organic or natural mineral fertiliser may be necessary during the establishment phase.

Permaculture is a type of farming which uses the diversity, stability and resilience of natural ecosystems to grow crops and livestock, compared to the destructive, unnatural single crops of monocultures, which require pesticides and fertilisers to function. Choose permaculture methods to grow your own organic food in nourishing, nutrient-dense soil, which can recycle waste, keep pests at bay and create a healthy habitat for wildlife.

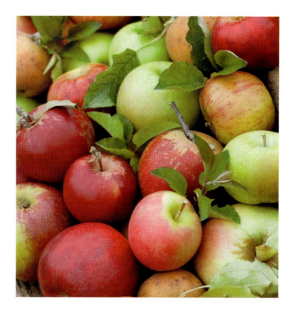

Avoid genetically modified foods

Genetic modification (GM) is a technology that takes genes from one life form and introduces them into another. Genes from bacteria, viruses, plants and animals are inserted into crops such as soybeans, canola, corn and cotton to grow commercially viable crops. Growing scientific evidence shows that GM crops are harmful to the environment and to human health. Buying organic ensures your food is free of genetic modification and irradiation.

Choose irradiation-free foods

Food irradiation exposes food to a source of radiation. It is used to destroy the unwanted pests that can accompany food when it is traded regionally or imported from other countries. Herbs, spices and tea are commonly irradiated foods. There are many problems with irradiation. It can mask spoiled food, kill good bacteria and encourage the growth of bad bacteria, devitalise and denature food, and impair flavour and cause chemical changes that are harmful to the consumer. A package of food that has been irradiated, or food that contains irradiated ingredients or components, must be labelled as such, but choosing organic can guarantee your food is not irradiated.

Choose chemical- and hormone-free

Industrial agriculture uses a variety of different chemicals to destroy pests and nourish the soil. Pesticides are used to prevent, destroy and repel pests. Fertilisers supply nutrients essential to the growth of plants but synthetic types cannot replicate the natural synergy of nutrients found in organic material such as blood and bone, compost, seaweed and manure. This can lead to the depletion of nutrients in our soil and therefore affect the quality of our food, as well as leave chemical residue in it.

Persistent organic pollutants (POPs) are the other types of chemicals found in our food chain. They originate from industrial pollution or are generated in natural processes such as bushfires. They are resistant to environmental degradation and can accumulate in human and animal tissue, and they have potentially significant impacts on human health and the environment. Dioxins are one type and are known as potent human carcinogens, endocrine disruptors, reproductive disruptors and immune disruptors.

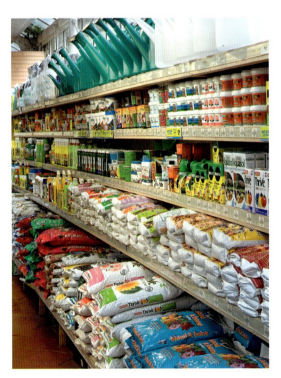

Hormones are found in our food chains as they are used by farmers to increase the productivity of certain types of cattle. Choosing food sourced from sustainable farming practices helps prevent hormones from ending up in our food chain.

Choose unprocessed food

Processing food can involve mechanical and chemical steps that alters or preserves it, or gives food a longer shelf life. Most people's perception of 'processing' is a negative one, especially when it applies to food. However, food processing can be good if food is prepared in a way that aids digestibility and preserves nutrients. Sometimes 'processing' simply means cooking, soaking or fermenting! The problem is that industrial food processing practices have developed that turn simple ingredients into nutrient-free or even harmful products rather than food.

Some problems with industrially processed foods are:

1. The natural nutrients are often destroyed.

2. Chemical or processed 'natural' additives are used.

3. Cheap, low-quality ingredients are used, which results in a cheap, low-quality food product.

4. Fast processing methods affect the quality of food, destroying valuable enzymes and nutrients.

5. Processing creates adverse cooking by-products such as acrylamide or advanced glycation end products (see explanation on page 29), which are detrimental to health.

6. Producers don't consider the fact that certain foods need to be prepared in ways to release antinutrients that may bind with or prevent uptake of other nutrients.

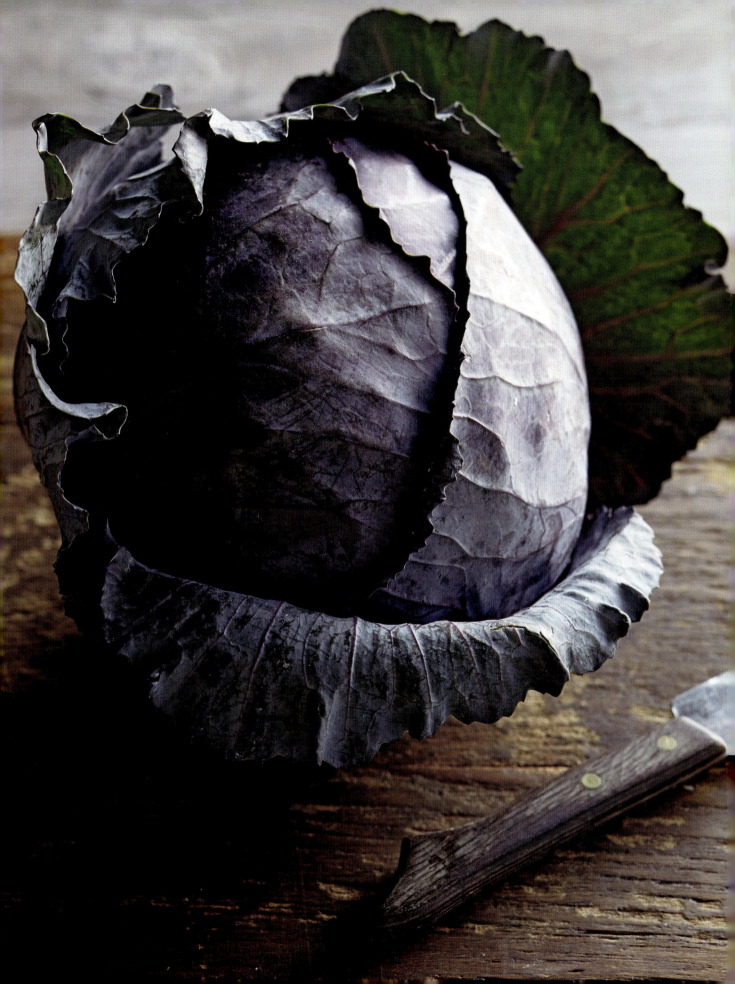

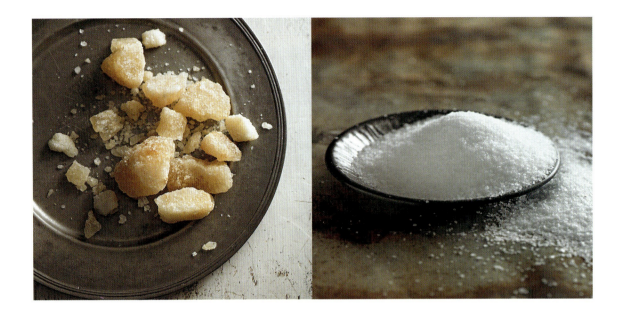

'Natural' doesn't always mean good
Natural ingredients are found in most food products. 'Natural' implies food that is minimally processed and has been produced using chemical-free methods. However, just because an ingredient is 'natural', it does not mean it is good for you, especially in large quantities – both sugar and salt could be considered natural ingredients, but they can be very harmful if eaten in excess. Apart from sugar (especially fructose) and salt, my top ingredients to watch out for and try to avoid are starch, 'vegetable' oils, soy lecithin, milk solids, white flour, soy flour and baker's yeast. Most of these are highly processed, meaning they've been stripped of nutrients and fibre and are often treated with all kinds of nasties such as bleach, which you really don't want to put in your body, and come from genetically modified crops.

Ten natural ingredients to avoid
1. Baker's yeast is used as a leavening agent. Although yeast can be fine for some people, it can contribute to various kinds of inflammation, leaky gut syndrome and yeast infections (candida), particularly if you have a compromised immune system.

2. High-fructose corn syrup is derived from corn, and is used as an alternative to sugar in processed food products because of its low cost and its high relative sweetness; it also, insidiously, allows a product to be marketed as 'sugar-free'. Studies have shown it to have even more detrimental effects than sugar because it is so highly processed. It is implicated in insulin resistance, diabetes, fatty liver and age-related diseases. It is very high in fructose; excessive fructose consumption can lead to fructose malabsorption, a condition similar to lactose intolerance, causing an array of digestive disorders.

3. Milk solids are spray-dried milk powder and are added to foods such as yoghurt or chocolate to give a creamy consistency and a thickening effect. The problem with milk solids is that the process used to produce it creates oxysterols, and these are thought to contribute to atherosclerotic plaques (the stuff coating the inside of the arteries that leads to heart disease).

4. Soy flour is used as an alternative to wheat flour because it has zero gluten content, but like soy lecithin it comes from highly processed industrial origins, as well as being a hormonal disruptor. See page 49 for more information.

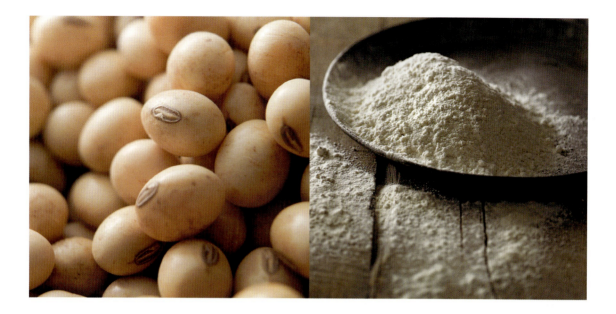

5. Soy lecithin is a natural emulsifier and stabiliser. The soy comes from a highly processed, industrially grown legume, often of GM origins. See page 19 for information on genetic engineering.

6. Starch is added to food in the highly processed form of maltodextrin, glucose syrup, dextrose, malitol, erythritol, sorbitol, mannitol and hydrogenated starch hydrolysate to sweeten, thicken and stabilise food. It has the same detrimental effects as sugar and high-fructose corn syrup.

7. Table salt is used as a flavour and preservative. It is a refined salt, containing about 97 per cent to 99 per cent sodium chloride, compared with the natural kinds, which contain many minerals. It usually contains an anti-caking agent: a chemical additive which makes it free-flowing. Salt, in its refined state, contributes to high blood pressure and oedema. Iodised salt is no better, as it is simply refined table salt with iodine.

8. Table sugar is used as a sweetener and preservative. It is highly refined compared to cane juice in its natural state. Sugar is very addictive and it is implicated in tooth decay, cravings, mood swings, increased appetite, energy highs and lows, diabetes, obesity, gout, heart disease and other age-related diseases.

9. Vegetable oils are derived from nuts, seeds and legumes, and are used as an ingredient in packaged food to give texture and flavour, and as a carrier for other flavours. They come from seeds produced by highly industrialised farming and processing methods. The common types are canola (also known as rapeseed), sunflower, safflower, grapeseed, rice bran, soybean, cottonseed, sesame, peanut and corn oil. This type of industrialisation yields more oil and is quicker to produce as well as giving greater stability in cooking and shelf life, but at the cost of detrimental consequences to our health. See pages 29–31 for processing methods to avoid.

10. White flour is used in baked goods, and it is not just stone-ground wheat. It is a highly refined cocktail. The bran and germ are removed and what's left is bleached white, then a maturing agent and preservatives are added to give the resulting product stability on the shelf and during cooking. Some are enriched with supplements or with a leavening agent (self-raising flour). Other white flours are derived from rice, corn or potato and undergo similar processing methods, yielding a highly refined, nutrient-devoid ingredient.

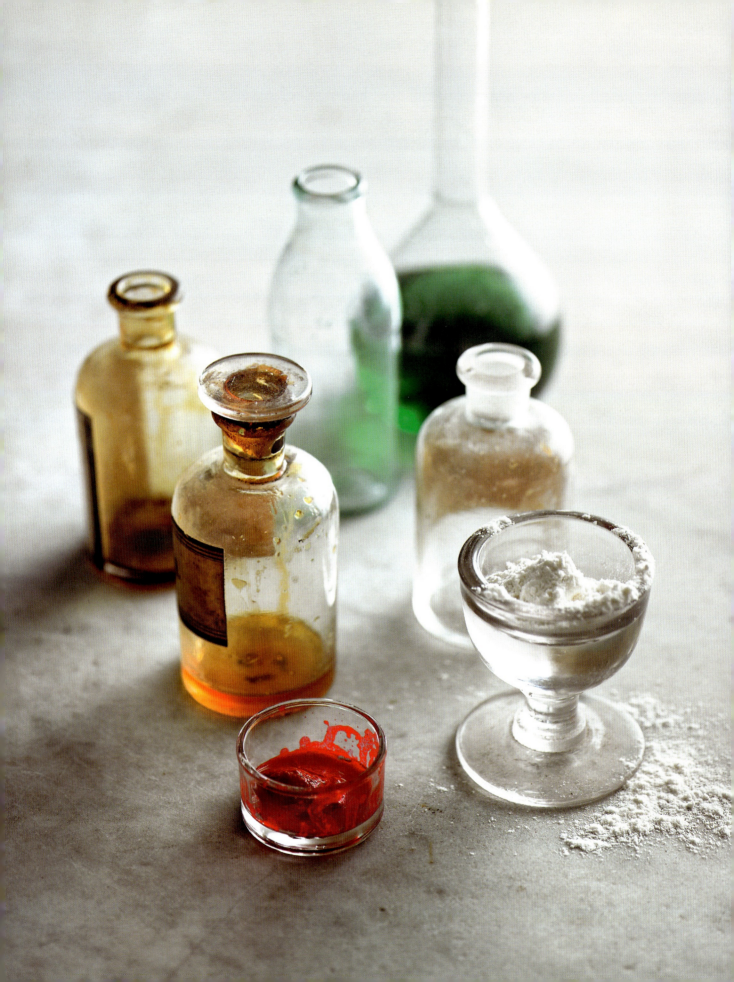

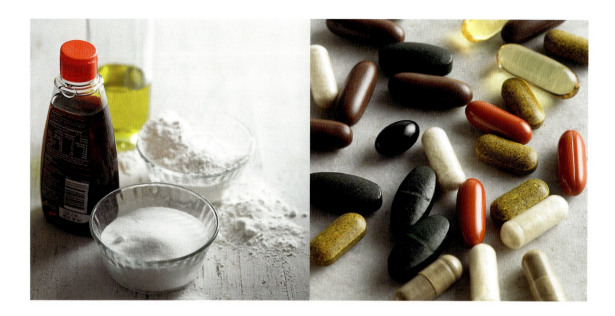

THE WHOLE TRUTH

The ingredients of ingredients do not legally have to be listed (for example, if a product contains tomato sauce, the individual ingredients of the sauce don't have to be mentioned). Neither does the processing method involved or the detrimental cooking by-products.

Ten chemical ingredients to avoid

Food additives are usually numbered with 'E' numbers rather than listing their full chemical names. Many food additives are linked with cancer, digestive problems, neurological conditions, ADHD, heart disease or obesity and more acute reactions such as hives or anaphylactic shock.

1. The agents No, not something from *The Matrix*, though you could be forgiven for thinking so. These include anticaking agents to stop salt or powdered foods from caking or sticking, antifoaming agents, glazing agents, flour treatment agents (often bleaches), humectanting agents and acidity regulators. Very often these are synthetic chemicals from dubious sources and can contribute to allergies or other physical problems.

2. Antibiotics are used by farmers to keep their animals free of diseases and, as a result, low residues of antibiotics may be present in some of the foods we eat. The widespread use of antibiotics inside and outside of medicine is playing a significant role in the emergence of antibiotic resistance. This means that bacteria can survive despite antibiotic doses that were previously effective. Outside medicine, antibiotics are fed to us through our food, such as farmed salmon.

3. Emulsifiers are used to bind two unblendable substances such as oil and water. Homogenised milk, for example, uses an emulsifier to disperse the cream, which would otherwise rise naturally to the top, throughout the milk. Natural emulsifiers include egg yolk, honey and soy lecithin. Sodium stearoyl lactylate (SSL) is an emulsifier for fat-in-water emulsions and also functions as a humectant to help the product retain moisture; it's commonly found in baked goods, desserts, chewing gum and toppings. Many additives such as SSL are classed as non-toxic. I believe the problem is that processed additives have a cumulative effect in the body, and as previously mentioned, the ingredients of ingredients are not listed so you won't necessarily know they're in your food. SSL production undergoes processing methods that include chemicals.

4. Food acids may be naturally or synthetically derived; they are added to make flavours 'sharper', and also as preservatives and antioxidants. Citric acid is one such example. It can damage tooth enamel as most of it is produced from corn sugar. Another is ascorbic acid, also known as vitamin C, which when consumed in unnatural amounts can also cause dental erosion and diarrhoea, and is linked to kidney stones.

5. Food colours may be added to food to replace those lost during preparation and make it look more attractive. Colour retention agents are used to preserve a food's existing colour. Some colours, such as carmine (E120) come from natural sources (the cochineal insect), but the process of extracting them involves such methods as boiling the dried insects in ammonia. Ugh. All artificial food colours are highly processed – give them a miss and try beetroot, for example, if you want to colour something pink.

6. Food flavourings and enhancers are additives that give food a particular taste or smell, and may be derived from natural ingredients or created artificially. Artificial ones can come from surprising sources such as crude oil or coal tar. Even if it's called a 'natural flavour', it is a highly processed ingredient used to flavour a processed food product. Real food is full of real flavour and no additives are required.

7. Functional ingredients are added to a food to create a new product with a new function, such as a health-promoting benefit; for example, foods fortified with supplements. Antioxidants such as vitamin C act as preservatives by inhibiting the effects of oxygen on food, and may be beneficial to health. The problem is that anything fortified with supplements has undergone a lot of processing, which destroys the natural nutrients and creates detrimental by-products. When lost nutrients are replaced with synthetic ones, the resulting product is devoid of the unique synergy of natural nutrients, enzymes and constituents which make our food vital, easily digested and assimilated. The sum of the parts does not equal the original whole.

8. Sweeteners are used instead of sugar. They can be naturally sourced, such as stevia, but are usually highly processed or artificial, such as aspartame, sucralose, neotame, cyclamates and saccharin. Stevia leaf is naturally green, but what we find in most health food stores is a processed, artificial version: a white powder or tablet, or a clear liquid. Artificial sweeteners have been associated with many health problems from diarrhoea to cancer and some research has shown they trigger the release of insulin just as sugar does. Artificial sweeteners are just that, artificial, and best avoided whether they're used to replace sugar or are found in processed, packaged ingredients.

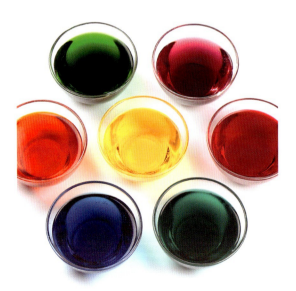

9. Synthetic preservatives are now used in many foods. Traditionally, food was preserved by using salt, rosemary extract, sugar, vinegar or alcohol, or by pickling, smoking and fermenting, but now, food manufacturers take the quick route and use chemicals. Unfortunately, a lot of people are allergic to these chemicals and can have quite alarming reactions to eating them, such as their throats swelling up, difficulty breathing, and hives.

10. Thickeners are additives derived from starches, vegetable gums, pectin, or proteins or synthetic chemicals. They increase the viscosity of a food product as well as stabilising and emulsifying ingredients. Large quantities can inhibit the absorption of some nutrients or cause stomach upsets. Those derived from starches contribute to the same diseases that are caused by sugar.

Other foods to avoid: Protein powders, bars and meal replacements

Protein powders are used as bodybuilding supplements and meal replacements in order to increase muscle growth, fat loss and improve athletic performance. I consider protein powders, whether the source is natural such as whey, pea or soy protein, or made from synthetic amino acids, to be highly processed, with added synthetic supplements. Protein powders are not complete foods, and are not highly digestible or easily assimilated, and can cause toxin build-up and vitamin or mineral toxicity or deficiencies. They are also devoid of natural fats, which assist in the assimilation of protein, or if they contain fats, they are usually highly processed and oxidised which contributes to inflammation. Eat real meat and eggs; try an 'Old-fashioned egg flip' – see page 81.

Protein bars are processed food bars packed with protein powders. They are low in calories and touted as being healthy snack foods for morning or afternoon tea. However, I believe they are best avoided for the same reasons as processed protein powders.

Meal replacements are totally unnecessary. Why isn't real food enough? The idea behind them is that they are portion controlled and calorie restricted. The problem is they are highly processed for preservation and are poorly sourced from both processed natural ingredients as well as many chemical additives. Read the ingredients on the packs. These are not healthy food replacements. Just eat sustainable, conscious, healthy food.

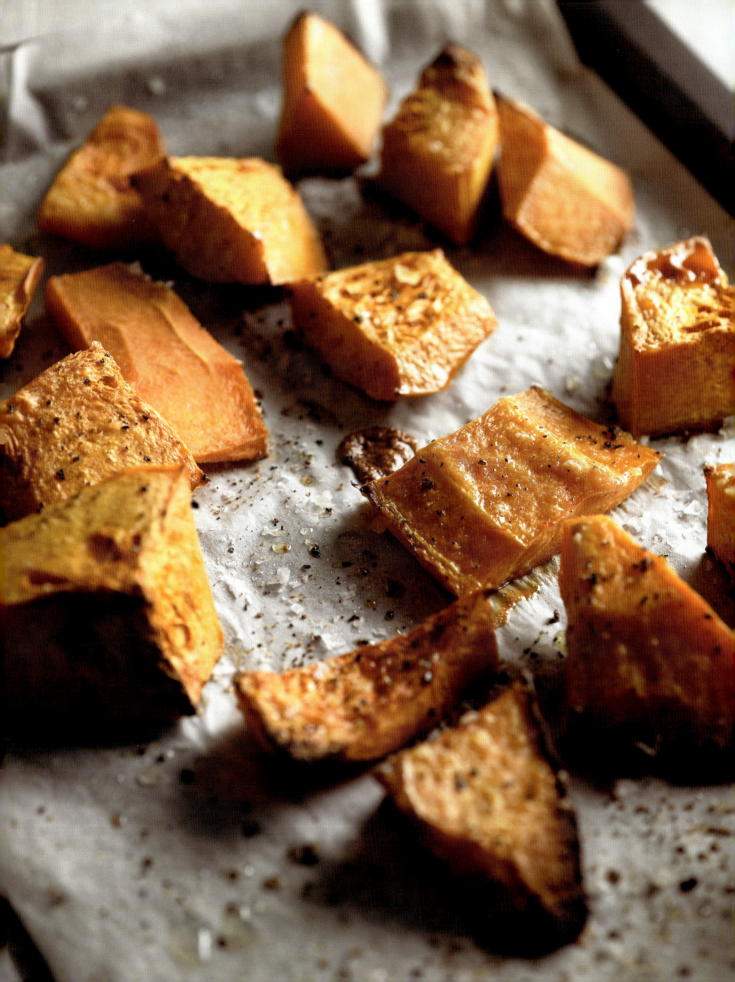

Cooking your food

Many foods need to be cooked before you can eat them; however, you need to be careful about which cooking methods you use as some are more harmful than others. You particularly need to watch out for cooking methods that cause the Maillard Reaction (MR), the name given to what happens when food browns as it's heated. The Maillard Reaction also occurs naturally in the human body as we age. Generally, MRs may play a role in some of the effects of ageing and some clinical complications of diabetes. MR end products, such as acrylamide, may also be toxic or carcinogenic.

Advanced glycation end products are also formed as part of the MR naturally in the body as we age. They are also produced by heating and cooking. They have been found to lead to age and diabetes-related chronic inflammatory diseases.

Polycyclic aromatic hydrocarbons are also formed by cooking. They are known to be carcinogenic and an industrial pollutant and high levels are found in meat cooked at high temperatures, especially when fat and juices from grilled meat drip on to the fire, causing flames. They are also formed in smoked fish.

Heterocyclic amines are also formed at high temperatures when cooking meat, seafood, poultry or pork at high temperatures. They are also carcinogenic.

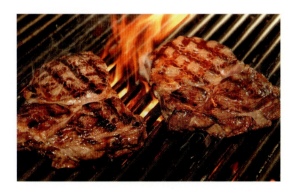

Ten cooking and processing methods to avoid

1. Frying

The problem with frying, particularly deep-frying, is that it produces toxic by-products due to the high temperature of the oil and often the type of oil or fat used – usually a processed transfat vegetable oil (see page 30).

The invention of non-stick cookware meant that you could fry with minimal or zero oil or fat but this also has its downfalls. The chemical coating on the pan can scratch off and end up in our food. One of the chemicals, called perfluorooctanoic acid (PFOA), is a known carcinogen. Stainless steel or cast iron is better. Avoid wok-fried or high-temperature stir-fries, especially meat with sugary sauces, as this causes the Maillard Reaction.

2. Grilling, barbecuing, and high-temperature baking or roasting

Grilling and barbecuing involves direct heat and can expose food to temperatures often in excess of 260°C, creating the Maillard Reaction and adverse cooking by-products. Barbecuing with the lid closed can be particularly dangerous to your health as toxic smoke, caused by meat fat dripping on coals, can infuse the meat.

Baking and roasting can also have these effects if the temperature is above 120°C. Avoid foods that have been cooked until browned or charred, and well-done meat unless it is slow-cooked at a low temperature. If you want medium or well-done steaks, sear them for one to two minutes on each side and then bake in the oven at a low temperature. Avoid factory-baked goods such as cereals, biscuits, chips and crackers, as these will also have been cooked at high temperatures.

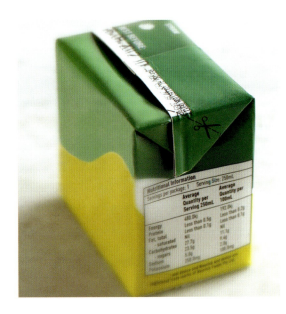

3. Ultraheating

Ultraheating or UHT is a method used to sterilise food by heating it at very high temperatures (over 135°C) for a short period. Long-life products are ultraheated. They include soy milk, rice milk, oat milk, cow's milk and juices, yoghurt, soups and wine. UHT gives food long life but this process can also cause the Maillard Reaction and adverse cooking by-products.

4. Fortification

If food is described as 'fortified', it means that nutrients (most commonly folic acid, iodine, fluoride or vitamin D) have been added to packaged foods such as cereals, breads, milk and milk products, fats and oils, beverages, protein powders and infant formulas. This is usually done because nutrients are lost in the manufacturing process; however, the added nutrients are synthetic and are not readily absorbed by the body.

5. Pasteurisation

Pasteurisation is the process of heating foods or drinks, such as milk and milk products, juice, soup, jam and sauces to give them a longer shelf life and greater stability. These foods are heated to 72°C for 15–20 seconds. The problem is not only are valuable micro-organisms destroyed (good bacteria), so are the natural enzymes and nutrients that aid digestion and prevent allergies. An example is raw goat milk, which I have found in my clinical practice to be an easier milk to digest and consume than pasteurised cow's milk, with little or no impact on sensitivities.

6. Homogenisation

The fat in milk normally separates and collects at the top. When milk is homogenised, it is forced at high pressure through small holes to make it consistent and uniform. The combination of shear forces and frictional heating of the milk during processing has many negative effects on its enzymes, microbes, fat globules and proteins.

Unhomogenised milk is available and is the better choice when purchasing milk.

7. Hydrogenation and interesterification

Avoid hydrogenated, partially hydrogenated and interesterified vegetable fats and oils in cooking or found in food products. The process of hydrogenation creates transfats, which have been found to have strong links to heart disease, diabetes, Alzheimer's, cancer, obesity, infertility, liver dysfunction and depression. They are predominantly found in convenient fast food, junk food, baked goods, shortenings and confectionery.

Interesterification With growing public awareness of the relationship between transfats, heart disease and other diseases, and the call for transfat-free products, industrial food processors had to come up with a new method. Interesterification is the processing method that has taken its place. This method is similar to partial or full hydrogenation in that it converts liquid oils into a harder substance that is used in margarines, shortenings, baked goods and confectionery. A chemical catalyst

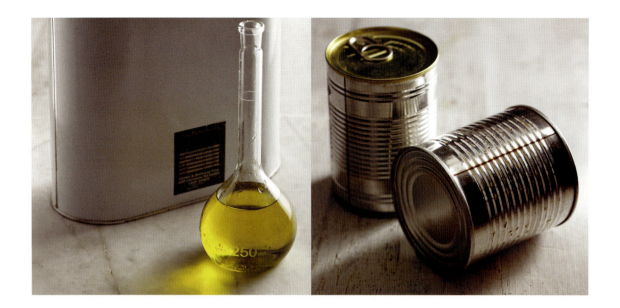

or enzyme is used, then the fat is neutralised, bleached and deodorised, all at high temperatures. The resulting product may be transfat-free, but it will still contain chemical residues, hexanes and many dangerous breakdown products.

Interesterified or hydrogenated vegetable oils are best avoided. Check carefully for them as an ingredient found in packaged foods and take-away food.

8. Chemical extraction

Vegetable oils are often extracted using solvent chemicals rather than the slower, more expensive cold-pressing method. The chemical that's most often used is petroleum-derived hexane, which is just as inedible as it sounds! You don't want that ending up in your food. Clear studies showing a direct link with hexane found in oils causing toxicity are not easy to find but hexane toxicity found in other products has been documented extensively as contributing to nervous and muscular system disorders. Always choose cold-pressed oils, and be aware that food products containing oils and fats are chemically extracted unless they state otherwise.

9. Canning

Canning is a method of preserving food. It undergoes high heat processes, refined salts are added for further preservation and the inside plastic lining of the can usually contains bisphenol A (BPA), an oestrogen mimicker that disrupts hormonal balance.

10. Microwaving

A microwave oven heats food by bombarding it with electromagnetic radiation. Like any high-temperature cooking method, it destroys the nutrients as well as creating toxic cooking by-products.

Microwaving has been shown to cause the greatest decrease in all studied antioxidants in broccoli, compared to other cooking methods such as steaming. A study has shown that microwaving garlic for just sixty seconds has a negative impact on its anticancer properties.

Powerwatch, a small non-profit, independent organisation with a central role in the UK Electromagnetic Field and Microwave Radiation health debate, says that even when the microwave oven is working correctly, the radiation levels within the kitchen are likely to be significantly higher than those from any nearby cellular phone base stations.

Remember also that electromagnetic radiation will travel through walls if the microwave oven is against an inside wall. There are also concerns that when packaged foods such as popcorn are microwaved, toxins from the plastic packaging can leak into the food.

How to stop using your microwave
This will take a little extra time and thought but will be well worth it for your health's sake! To reheat food, put it with a little water in a pan or pot, stir and put lid on, then heat through gently. To defrost food, place it in your fridge and allow to gently thaw out over a day. To make oat porridge, soak oats in water, some lemon juice and natural salt in a pot overnight. The next day, add more water or milk and stir on stovetop until creamy and cooked.

Ten food preparation methods to choose

The best methods of preparing food aim to simply enhance what is already naturally there. Doing this aids digestion, brings out natural flavour, preserves valuable nutrients and is better for you. And quite simply, it's so much more pleasant to eat food made with love, care and respect for where the ingredients come from and the people and animals that produced it.

These methods are based on gentle, slow cooking and low to medium temperatures. Healthy food preparation methods allow the ingredients to reign supreme. It's great to see that traditional food preparation methods are making a full return after years of absence due to our busy, stressed-out lifestyles. We are still busy but I believe we are reprioritising and making our health come first.

We are what we eat and we eat what we are. Often clients come to me with their minds and bodies dying of malnutrition. As we move back into our kitchens to create nourishing foods we come back to ourselves and remember the pleasure and goodness of eating home-cooked meals.

1. Steaming
Steaming allows food to be gently cooked without burning, overcooking or using processed fat or vegetable oil. Use a steamer or simply add an inch of water to a pot, add vegetables and put lid on. Serve with high-quality olive oil or butter, natural salt and a squeeze of lemon.

2. Simmering
Every culture has their traditional soup for healing or as a starter before a meal. Common to them all is the process of simmering some combination of meat, vegetables and water in a pot until cooked.

3. Braising or stewing
These methods produce good old-fashioned comfort food. Long, drawn-out flavours and warm homely aromas are created from slow cooking at low temperatures.

Braises generally use cubed meat or small cuts with the bone in, such as lamb shanks. A braise uses very little liquid in relation to the quantity of meat.

Stews use more liquid and takes less time to cook as the meat is completely submerged.

4. Pan-frying or gentle sauteing
Pan-frying is a gentle way of cooking food in a pan or pot without the use of much fat or oil. Use this method for fillets of meat.

Sauteing uses higher temperatures but for health purposes and to avoid burning food, keep temperatures no higher then a medium heat. Saute vegetables and cubed meats and fish.

The best fats for pan-frying or sauteing include: tallow (beef fat), lard (pig fat), duck or goose fat, coconut oil, butter, cold-pressed olive oil (combined with butter) and ghee. All animal fats should be grass-fed and organic.

5. Casseroling
Casseroles are usually cooked slowly in a dish in the oven, often uncovered, so heat can circulate all around the cooking dish. They consist of pieces of meat or seafood

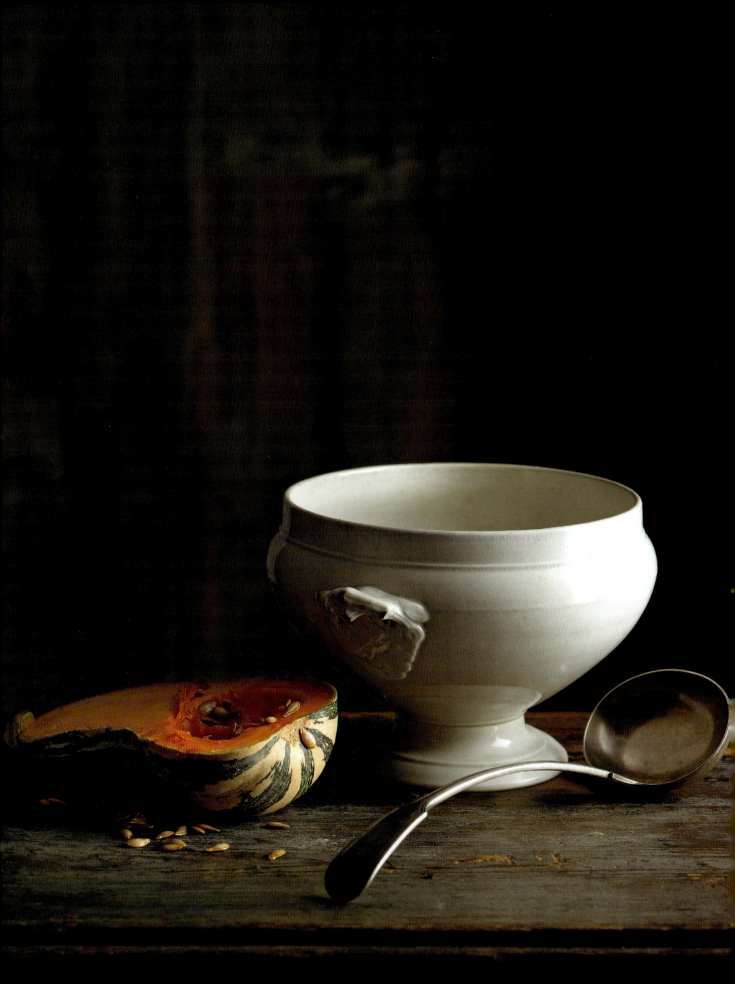

and chopped vegetables. Types of casseroles include ragout, hotpot, cassoulet, tagine, osso buco and stroganoff.

6. **Baking and slow roasting**
When baking, keep the oven as low as you can (see Recipes section from page 76 onwards for specific details). Baking dishes made from stainless steel are best, lined with baking paper or coated well with butter or olive or coconut oil.

Slow roasting at low temperatures in the oven, 95°C–120°C, is best when cooking with large cuts of meat, whole chickens or root vegetables such as potatoes. Slow roasting creates less moisture loss and a more tender result, as more of the collagen that makes meat tough is dissolved.

7. **Eating food raw**
Raw food movements have been encouraged by vegans, vegetarians and people following the Paleolithic diet, based on the understanding that uncooked foods are in their most natural state, unaltered by processing and therefore more nutrient-dense. They are also based on the belief that the hunter-gatherer didn't own an oven, or have the hybrids of new food on offer. I believe that all nuts, seeds, grains and beans need to be prepared by soaking, sprouting and fermenting to aid digestion and enhance nutrition.

Certain vegetables and fruit are better when cooked, such as those containing oxalates and goitrogens (see page 35, opposite). If you are thin, wiry, cold and suffer from a nervous disposition, cold raw foods are best avoided until you can transition to more robust health and wellbeing. Other than that, raw food is ideal. Enjoy raw eggs in old-fashioned egg flips (see page 81). Raw meats and fish in the form of tartare and ceviche are good, as are raw dairy products if you can find them.

8. **Soaking**
Soaking is a preparation step to make our nuts, seeds, grains and beans ready for cooking, sprouting or fermenting, which in turn makes them more digestible. Soaking in salt, water and an acid medium is most ideal. Refer to page 213 for soaking methods.

9. **Fermenting**
This is a food process which converts carbohydrates to alcohols, leavens bread or is used to produce lactic acid in sour foods such as sauerkraut, yoghurt or vinegar. Fermenting preserves foods, adds flavour, enhances nutrition and eliminates antinutrients.

10. **Sprouting**
Sprouting makes seeds, grains, beans and nuts alive with available nutrients. Essentially they are all seeds and to digest and access their nutrition we need to create an environment similar to damp, hot, humid soil, with sunlight and water to release a sprout. This is the life of the seed. Sprouting also releases antinutrients which bind to our minerals.

Antinutrients and why we need to soak, ferment, sprout and cook our foods

Antinutrients are substances found in food that bind to our nutrients and prevent us from absorbing them. Therefore, our food needs to be prepared in a way that gets rid of antinutrients or makes them more digestible.

Cyanogenic glycosides are found in plants such as wheat, corn, oats, peanuts and cassava. When the plant tissue is damaged, the toxin hydrogen cyanide is released. Humans can tolerate small amounts, but too much can be lethal. To minimise the amount of hydrogen cyanide that gets consumed, the cell walls of the plant need to be damaged (by chopping, grinding, cooking and so on) so that it is released harmlessly into the air.

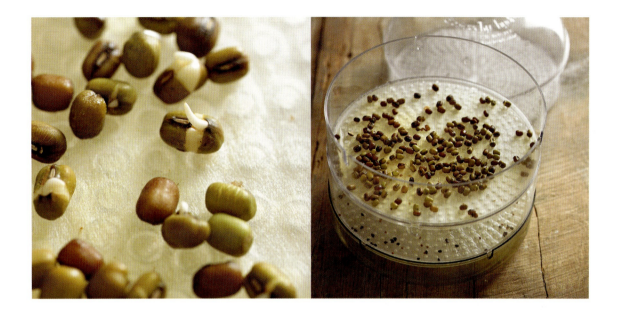

Goitrogens interfere with your ability to absorb iodine, a very important element for the function of your thyroid gland. Foods rich in goitrogens include but are not limited to soybeans, pine nuts, peanuts, millet, bamboo shoots and the brassica family of vegetables. Cooking inactivates goitrogens (except in the case of millet and soybeans, which need to be fermented).

Lectins are chemicals that are found in an active form in the mature seeds, tubers and sap of many common food plants, particularly the legume family. They can damage the walls of red blood cells and induce clumping. They are not very readily absorbed in the digestive tract, but can in some cases damage its cell walls and interfere with nutrient uptake and growth. Lectins are reduced by cooking.

Oxalates are soluble salts found in particularly high concentrations in rhubarb, spinach and unripe tomatoes. They are usually excreted in the urine, but if a lot are consumed, they can cause you to accumulate calcium in the urinary tract and make dietary calcium less available to your body. They can also bind to iron and prevent you from absorbing it. Oxalates are reduced by cooking.

Phytic acid binds to important minerals such as calcium, magnesium, iron and zinc. This causes them to become insoluble so they cannot be absorbed in the intestines. Phytic acid is found in the hulls of nuts, seeds and grains. Simply cooking your food goes some way towards reducing the phytic acid content, but even more effective is soaking them in an acid medium (eg water with a little lemon juice), lactic acid fermentation and sprouting.

Trypsin inhibitors are proteins which inhibit the action of the digestive enzyme trypsin, making it unable to break down and release amino acids to the body. Trypsin inhibitors can be found in legumes and can be deactivated by heating. Soy and lima beans are some examples of foods rich in trypsin inhibitors.

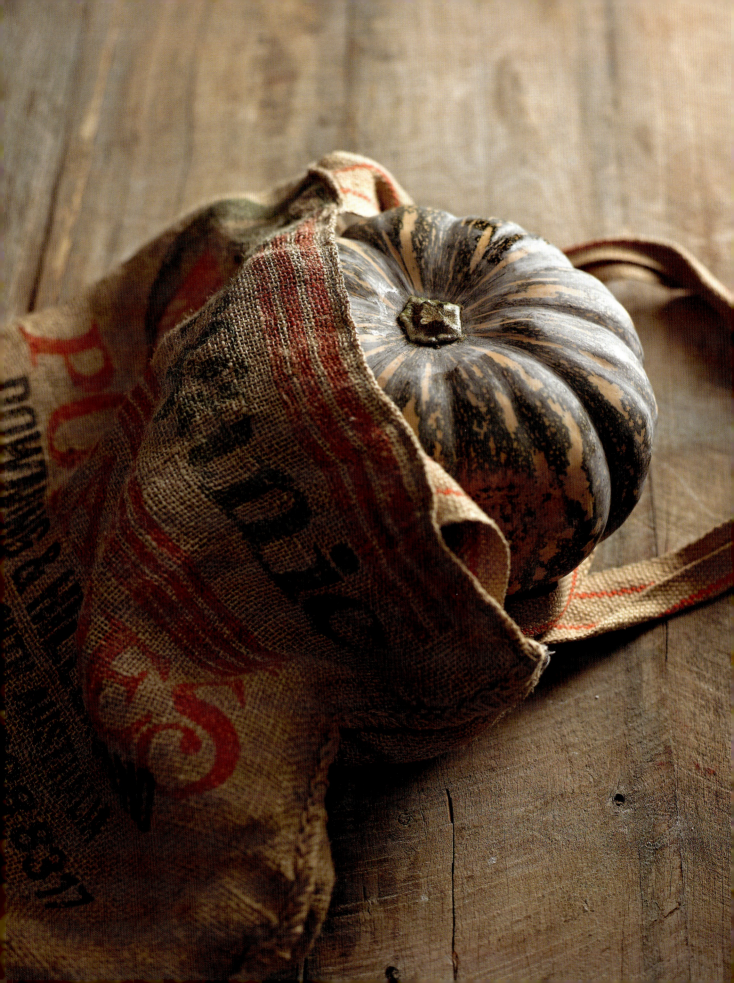

Choosing conscious, sustainable wholefood

Walking through the supermarket, convenience store or health food store aisle is no doubt confusing. There are so many choices and varieties of the same foods. Apply these simple rules during your next shopping trip to make the process of choosing the best foods simple and convenient.

1. No matter what the food or drink, always consider the source, processing and preparation principles I have outlined.
2. Read labels well, particularly the ingredients; learn more about the brand and their source of ingredients and if you are still unsure, then a general rule is, if it is in a packet and is ready-to-eat food, it is best avoided. One example is cereal. If it is a single ingredient, such as quinoa, then it is acceptable as long as the ingredient is in its whole state.
3. Buy your meat from a pastured butcher, bread from a sourdough bakery, seafood from the markets, and dairy products, eggs, vegetables, fruit, oils, fats and dried goods from an organic farmers' market or a reputable organic health food store.
4. Look for certification labels such as organic or biodynamic, humane and ethical.
5. Get to know your retailer or food supplier. Ask questions and do your own research.

Vegetables and fruit
Choose organic, biodynamic or chemical-free. Choose seasonal and local. Many markets chop off the tops of vegetables, especially beets and fennel. Ask if you can keep them, and save them for stocks, or steam and add olive oil and lemon juice and season well. Prewashed and cut, ready-to-eat vegetables in bags or plastic containers, such as lettuces or stock vegetables such as carrots, celery and onion, do offer convenience but you're paying extra money for plastic you're just going to throw away. Choose fruit and vegetables in their whole state because this preserves their nutrients and they undergo less processing and preparation. Grow as much as you can on your balcony or in your garden. Become part of a community garden.

Frozen vegetables and fruit are precut for convenience or are found in their whole state in the form of berries. Vegetables such as peas are boiled or blanched for a few minutes before they are frozen. The jury is out on whether there are differences in nutritional value between fresh and frozen vegetables. The most important factor is that your produce comes from a quality, organic and biodynamic source.

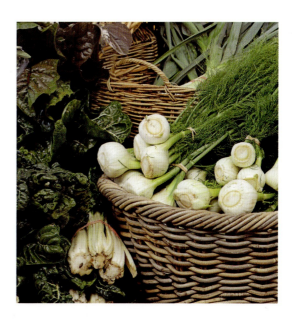

GENERAL PRINCIPLES – FOOD FOR LIFE

Dried fruit The problem with dried fruit is firstly that it often contains artificial preservatives, and secondly that you would never eat this amount of fresh fruit in one sitting. Sulphur dioxide is a common preservative found in dried fruit which protects its colour and flavour. This is most obviously seen with dried apricots. Those without sulphur dioxide are brown while those with this preservative are orange. This preservative can induce asthma in those who are susceptible. Vegetable oil instead of sulphites may be used to preserve dried fruits. Glycerine or another sweetener such as sugar or juice concentrate may also be added as a preservative and, obviously, to add more sweetness. Sometimes synthetic anticlumping agents are also added to prevent fruit from sticking together.

Dried fruit is full of fructose and can create sugar highs and lows. If you choose to eat or cook with it, rehydrate it in water for a couple of hours and avoid those with additives.

Pickles

A pickle is usually a vegetable that has been preserved by anaerobic fermentation in brine, to produce lactic acid, or in an acid solution, such as vinegar. Pickling can preserve perishable foods or foods to be enjoyed in another season for months.

Make sure pickles or cultured vegetables contain straightforward ingredients, such as natural salt, fresh or dried herbs and spices, and quality vinegar if vinegar is used. Better still, make your own. Refer to the recipes on page 221.

Meat

When buying meat, whether it be beef, lamb or pork, the most important consideration is whether it came from a healthy pastured animal. Make sure it is grass-fed or pastured and grass-finished. Choose a variety of cuts with bones, cartilage and fat. Eat the organs and keep the bones for stocks – both provide you with essential nutrients. Red meat has significantly more B12, iron, and zinc than white meat and a healthier fatty acid profile. The fat of ruminants comprises approximately equal parts of saturated and monounsaturated fat, with only a small amount of polyunsaturated fat.

Chicken is often intensively farmed, unless it comes from a small, sustainable and environmentally conscious farmer. I prefer to eat less chicken (and always whole) and more beef, lamb, pork and seafood instead. 'Boiler' hens, usually egg layers, offer the best flavour and mineral nutrition for stocks as they are older (usually one year old) and have more developed bones, compared to the soft bones of a 'broiler'.

Deli meats should be ones that are preserved traditionally by curing with salt, sugar, spices or smoking. Salt retards the growth of microorganisms; sugar feeds healthy microorganisms and balances the saltiness, especially in bacon and ham. Nitrates are also used to preserve deli meats. The jury is out on whether they are bad for you – some believe they are carcinogenic. Ham off the bone is cured pork leg. Pork was traditionally dry cured, rubbed with a salt mixture, then smoked and left to

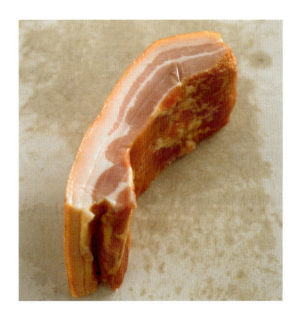

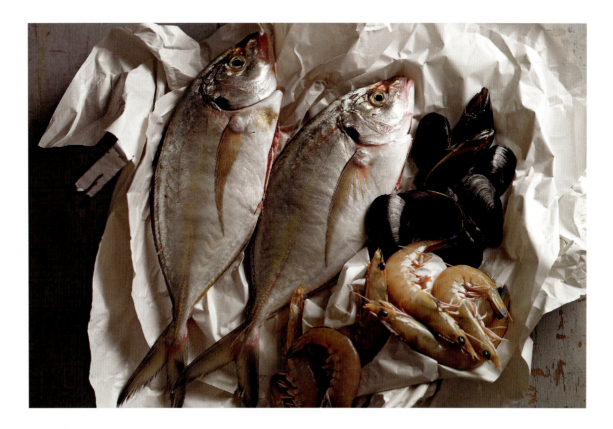

slowly air-dry and mature to preserve it for long periods. Today, it's usually wet cured, which means it's treated with a salt- and sugar-based solution before cooking. This faster process makes it moister and less salty, but it has a shorter shelf life than the dried, cured ham, and it also contains sugar.

Seafood

Sustainable seafood is fish and shellfish caught with minimal impact on fish populations and marine environments. Avoid precooked frozen fish as they are usually full of processed ingredients and not as nutrient-dense as fresh fish or well-cooked seafood at home.

According to Greenpeace, most tuna sold in Australia is still caught using destructive fishing methods, which obliterate tuna stocks and kill other marine life, such as dolphins. This has to stop in order to restore the health of our oceans. Apart from how they catch the fish and prepare it, consider the additives that are added to your tuna; for example, rancid oils, refined salts and flavour additives and preservatives. Also consider the canning process, which applies heat that destroys the natural oils in fish, particularly omega 3, and the lining of the can, which is detrimental to our health.

Humans are responsible for the toxins contaminating seafood through environmental pollution. These include heavy metals, such as mercury and lead, and industrial chemicals like dioxins and pesticides. These usually enter the marine environment from industrial agriculture and are found in the highest concentrations in those animals that are high up the food chain such as sharks and swordfish. Food Standards Australia and New Zealand (FSANZ) also recommends avoiding orange roughy and catfish in addition to shark and swordfish.

Dairy products

It is said that humans are the only species that drink another mammal's milk. Lactose intolerance is a common problem; I believe it is usually due to poorly sourced and highly processed milk from unhealthy, grain-fed cows. Repairing digestive function and establishing healthy micro-flora in the gut seems to help milk digestion, as well as consuming milk in its unprocessed state. This is something I have seen in my practice over nearly two decades. There are, however, some clients who, even after restoring good health and introducing unprocessed milk into their diets, still experience lactose intolerance.

Genetics also seems to play a role. The enzyme lactase, which is located in the small intestine, is responsible for digestion of lactose in milk. You produce a lot of lactase during infancy, but in most mammals, including many humans, this declines after the weaning phase. In other healthy humans, lactase activity persists at a high level throughout adult life, enabling them to digest lactose as adults. This dominantly inherited genetic trait is known as lactase persistence. Multiple studies indicate that whether or not you keep producing enough lactase to digest milk as an adult is genetically programmed.

Milk is milk. It should come from an animal, not a grain, bean, nut or seed. Choose whole fat and unhomogenised milk that comes from pastured animals. Goats' milk is legally sold as a raw milk in Australia, but cow's milk unfortunately has to be pasteurised by law. Avoid lactose-free milk, lite, diet, enriched milk or milk that is ultra heated or uses aseptic processing and packaging, for example long-life packs.

Yoghurt is best when it's made from full-fat milk from healthy pastured cows. Avoid ones with milk solids or milk powder which is added to give yoghurt a creamy consistency. Even the best, well-sourced yoghurts contain milk solids. Yoghurt is best bought plain, made from real milk (not soy) fermented with natural cultures or probiotics and set in the tub or container. You can also make your own from organic milk; see the recipe on page 218. Add your own fruit for flavour, spices such as vanilla or cinnamon and natural sweetness from organic green leaf stevia or a very small amount of honey.

Cheese is also best made from full-fat milk sourced from healthy pastured animals. Commercial cheeses are made with fresh milk or milk powder, emulsifiers, refined salts, preservatives, and food colouring. Traditional cheese is made by adding a starter culture (bacteria) to milk, then rennet which coagulates the milk; this then produces curds and whey which are separated and salted. The curds are pressed and left to mature depending on what cheese is being made. Simple!

Oils and fats

Oils and fats are used for cooking and as a food ingredient in packaged foods. For the simple purpose of knowing the good and not so good types, let's categorise them as animal fats and plant fats.

Normally we are told that saturated fats, which include all the animal fats, are not good for us. True if they are poorly sourced (from grain-fed, unhealthy animals) or derived from

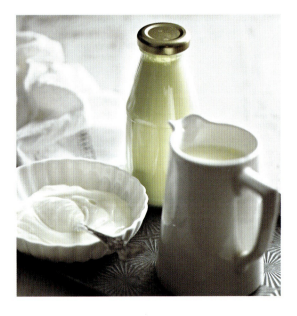

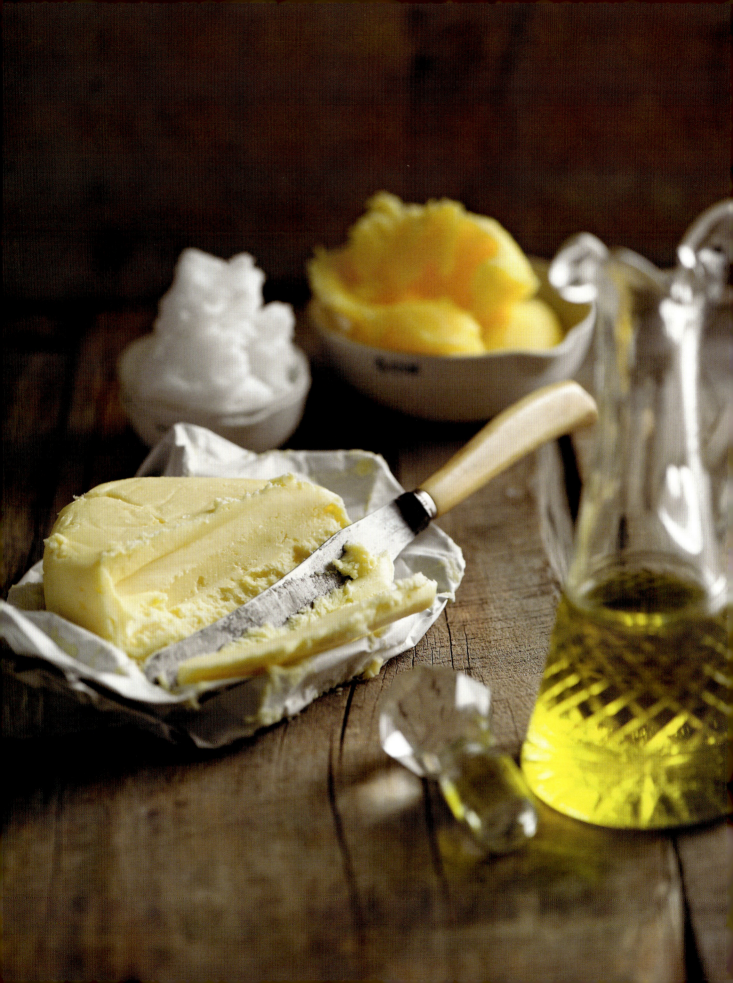

highly processed cooking methods. Not true if from grass-fed or pasture-finished animals, non-farmed seafood, whole dairy and whole eggs, all of which are sources of beneficial and essential fats such as omega 3, which is an anti-inflammatory; fat-soluble vitamins A, D and K2, which are essential for mineral absorption and healing and repair; and healthy saturated fats, which contain healthy cholesterol for brain and nerve function, cell membrane health, and help your body make vitamin D and bile acid (which you need to be able to digest fats). They also provide all those essential hormones to help your reproductive system to function, regulate your blood sugar, balance the minerals in your body, and regulate your blood pressure and adrenal glands.

Saturated cooking oils and fats are stable as long as temperatures are kept below 120°C. Make sure your fish oils are fermented or cold extracted and from sustainable and healthy fish.

Read labels carefully – most cod liver oils and fish oils available worldwide are molecularly distilled, a process that heats the oil and strips away most of the naturally occuring nutrients. On the other hand, fermented cod liver oil is not molecularly distilled. Produced using the age-old technique of lacto-fermentation, it is a completely raw product, rich in enzymes and associated nutrients. This makes it an amazing and unique food, untouched by modern processing methods and as a result, it is extremely stable and easily absorbed by your body. I recommend the Green Pasture brand.

Plant fats These are sourced from seeds, nuts or beans and may also be called vegetable oils. Normally we are told all unsaturated fats – ie most vegetable oils and vegetable fats – are good for us. But this is not true and too general. They are not good for us if they are poorly sourced (from industrial agriculture) and highly processed (chemically extracted, high heat method applied, hydrogenated or interesterified – see pages 30–31). They are

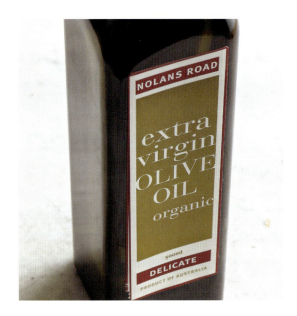

susceptible to oxidative damage, which is a risk factor for several modern diseases, including heart disease.

Choose oils that are produced by sustainable agricultural methods and cold-pressed types such as coconut oil and olive oil. Note that extra virgin (first pressed) is the best. Coconut oil is rich in saturated fats and is a more stable plant fat when cooking as long as temperatures are kept below 120°C. Olive oil is best combined with butter or used at low to medium temperatures. Good-quality olive oil and coconut oil will solidify in the fridge. If they remain liquid when cold or have no scent, they are refined or processed. Olive oil has a long history of study and research, as it is part of a healthy Mediterranean diet that protects the heart, amongst other benefits. Coconut oil is also well researched for its benefits in fat loss, digestive health and anti-microbial properties as well as protecting the heart. Flaxseed oil is touted as an essential, healthy oil that supplies omega 3, but it's important to remember that if you are nutritionally deficient in other areas, your body will not be able to convert it to a form it can use. Omega 3 is an essential anti-inflammatory fat. It is very unstable and tends to oxidise with heat and light, so if you are taking flaxseed oil it needs to be kept in the fridge.

Nuts and seeds

Like vegetable oils, nuts and seeds such as almonds, macadamias, pecans, walnuts and brazil nuts, and sunflower seeds, pepitas, linseed/flaxseed and sesame seeds should be limited or moderated because of the high levels of omega-6 fats that many of them contain. Omega 6 is pro-inflammatory and reduces the beneficial omega 3.

Commercial types are normally roasted, old, rancid (oxidised), coated with refined salt and full of phytic acid (see page 35 on phytic acid/antinutrients). Buy whole raw nuts and seeds, then soak well in an acid medium (lemon juice, whey or vinegar), natural salt and filtered water, to make them digestible. You can also buy 'activated' nuts that have already been prepared well to rid them of phytic acid. Eat a very small handful a few times per week and avoid if you are nutrient-deficient in minerals as your body can accumulate phytic acid if you eat too many nuts, seeds, grains and beans whether prepared well or not. The best types are those without skin such as blanched almonds or macadamias (which can be consumed raw as it's the skin that contains the phytic acid).

Avoid pre-ground nuts and seeds as they are not fresh and already rancid. If you need almond meal for a recipe, grind it freshly yourself and use immediately or keep refrigerated. Avoid nut butters, which are often already oxidised and full of phytic acid. Note: phytates are not bad for everyone; they are useful for those with excess iron and can be used to bind iron in conditions such as haemachromatosis or reduce calcium kidney stones. Consult your health professional about what's right for you.

Herbs and spices

Herbs and spices are available in many forms: fresh, dried, powdered or as a paste. Fresh is always best when it comes to the leaves or aerial parts of a herb. Examples include basil, parsley and coriander leaf.

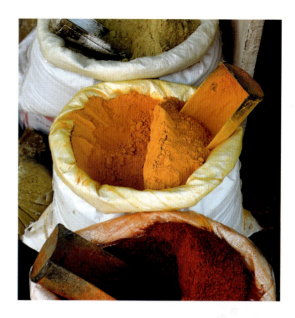

Dried herb leaves are more concentrated and are useful when a more intense flavour is required, such as in casseroles, stews, slow food cooking and soups. When it comes to a spice, the dried form is best, especially if the part used is the seed, pod, bark or twig. Examples include cinnamon, star anise, cardamom pods and aniseed.

Many herbs and spices are not grown in Australia. When we bring them into the country they need to be irradiated by law. Best to choose organic and Australian-grown, as this guarantees they are irradiation free. Organic also guarantees there are no chemicals added, such as pesticides.

Grains and pseudocereals

Grains are corn, wheat, rice, barley, spelt, millet, oats, sorghum and triticale. Pseudocereals are non-grasses that are used in much the same way as cereals/grasses or true grains. These include amaranth, quinoa and buckwheat. Grains come in many forms, such as flour, pasta, noodles, breads, cakes, biscuits, muesli bars, breakfast cereals and as an ingredient in many processed, packaged foods. Grains are only available in such great abundance due to industrial agriculture; our

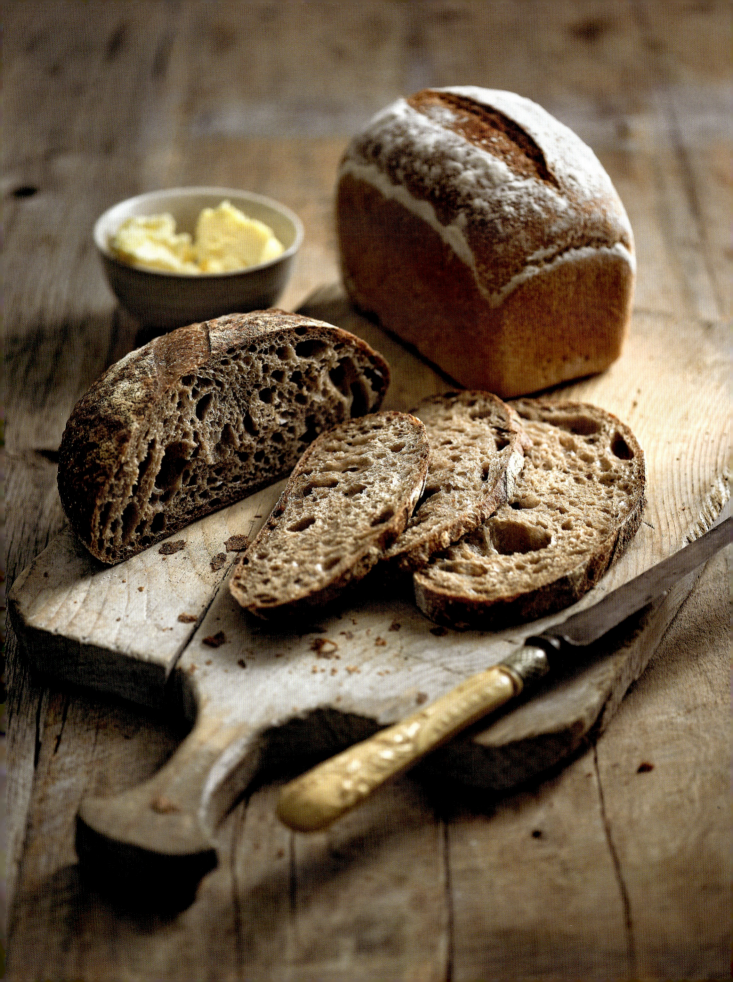

bodies are not made to eat large amounts of them. They are also full of antinutrient phytic acid.

Keep your grains to a minimum amount per week, one serve once or twice a week maximum, and make sure to prepare them well. Avoid them for periods of time and see how you feel, especially if you suffer digestive issues, inflammation, weight gain or an auto-immune condition. Most clients I see do better without grains.

Healthy breads are those that use well-sourced ingredients. Even so, keep consumption of these to a minimum per week, ensure they have no processed additives and are prepared in a way that deactivates the antinutrients, to make them more digestible. The best are sprouted or sourdough-fermented breads.

Sourdough bread is made from a sourdough starter, which is a symbiotic culture of bacteria and yeast present in a mixture of flour and water. This is used to ferment the flour, releasing antinutrients such as phytic acid which bind to calcium, magnesium, iron and zinc. This increases the nutrient density of the bread and makes it much easier to digest.

Sprouted bread is made from whole grains (rather than flour) that have been allowed to sprout; that is, to germinate. It is often eaten uncooked, or slightly heated. When grains, seeds and nuts are germinated, their nutritional content changes and, as they are generally not cooked, they retain their natural plant enzymes. These enzymes are beneficial for helping you digest the seeds and nuts and release the phytic acids.

The not-so-healthy breads are cooked by fast methods, such as quick chemical leavening or yeast leavening, which do not allow the grain to fully ferment. The consequences are poor digestion, bloating and a binding of valuable nutrients. They are also full of the natural and chemical additives I previously mentioned that should be avoided: bread improvers such as sodium metabisulfite, used to improve the texture and volume; refined salt, added to enhance flavour; vegetable oil, used to give flavour, stability and texture; flavourings, folic acid and other synthetic supplements; soya flour, used to 'improve' consistency; calcium propionate, used to inhibit mould growth; emulsifiers and stabilisers such as starch or anti-staling agents, all combined with a GM grain such as a wheat, soy or corn base.

Breakfast cereals, porridge and muesli All breakfast cereals, whether organic or not, are highly processed. The process can both denature the protein and gelatinise the starch. It will help deactivate antinutrients, making the cereal more digestible than raw grains, but it also creates insulin-desensitising starches, which are a risk factor for developing diabetes and also cause the product to lose nutrients.

The high temperatures alone destroy natural nutrients, and the resulting product is often then sprayed with dextrin, vegetable oil and sugar. Puffed grains, whether for cereals or rice cakes, are grains popped at such high temperatures that they destroy valuable nutrients.

Whole grain or pseudo cereals are best, prepared in a way that is digestible, such as Bircher-style muesli soaked in yoghurt or made into a porridge by soaking and cooking the next day. Flaked grains are not as good but are better than a cereal flake or puffed grain, as they are simply a wholegrain that is rolled out and flattened.

Cakes, biscuits, crackers and muesli bars Processed, ready-to-eat types of these products also contain most of the 'chemical and natural ingredients to avoid' I've described. They undergo high-temperature cooking, which creates toxic cooking by-products. Muesli bars and crackers are considered 'health foods' and are consumed as a guilt-free snack, but their sugar percentage alone is enough to make them unhealthy.

Constipation is not a fibre deficiency
Fibre is found naturally in well-prepared whole grains, legumes, nuts, seeds, vegetables and fruit. Did people have constipation before grains were produced on an industrial scale? The answer is no. Bran, the modern solution for constipation, is an indigestible food phytate and a waste by-product of refined flours and cereals. Hydration, healthy gut flora, plenty of wholefoods (vegetables, animal protein and fats), removing the reliance on caffeine and processed ingredients, and squatting and relaxation are the solution to healthy bowels.

Gluten is a protein found in some cereal grains: wheat (wheat is found also as burghul, semolina, couscous, farina, wheatgerm, wheat bran), oats, rye, barley, triticale, kamut and spelt. The gluten-free diet has quickly become one of the fastest growing nutritional movements in America, according to the National Foundation for Coeliac Awareness, partly because of increasing numbers of diagnoses of coeliac disease. Coeliac disease is an autoimmune digestive disease that damages the villi of the small intestine and interferes with the absorption of nutrients from food. Essentially, the body attacks itself every time a person with coeliac disease consumes gluten. You don't have to have coeliac disease to be gluten-intolerant though – a sensitivity to gluten is quite common. These individuals can also experience an array of symptoms if they eat gluten.

If you are avoiding gluten, try also to avoid ready-made or ready-to-eat gluten-free products. They are highly processed and usually made from highly refined gluten-free alternatives such as potatoes, corn, soybean and rice. They are simply devoid of nutrients because of the intense processing methods used, and are too high in starch.

Gluten-free grain alternatives include millet and rice or the pseudocereals (these are not really grains), such as amaranth, quinoa or buckwheat. Eat these in their whole state prepared well (through soaking, fermenting or sprouting).

Those who are true coeliacs might feel better eliminating grains altogether as gluten-containing grains may mix with gluten-free grains at the factory end and this is enough to cross-contaminate them with gluten.

GLUTEN IS CONTAINED IN MANY FOODS

1. Commercial soups and tinned products such as baked beans.
2. Sauces such as soy sauce.
3. Thickeners found in ice cream, custards, cheeses, creams and yoghurts.
4. Tapioca starch and icing sugar.
5. Pasta, most cereals, muesli, breads, biscuits, cakes, batters, crumbs and flours (unless specified), farina and thickeners, malt, soba and udon noodles, pumpernickel bread, pastry, pizza, pancakes, waffles, doughnuts, wafers, cones and rusks.
6. Sausages, burgers, rissoles, frozen dinners and imitation seafood.
7. Yeasted spreads such as Vegemite and Marmite.
8. Commercial condiments e.g. chutney, relishes, pickles, mustard, stock cubes and gravy mixes.
9. Coffee substitutes, drinking chocolate, beer, ale, lager, porter and stout.
10. Licorice, flavouring essences and filled chocolates.

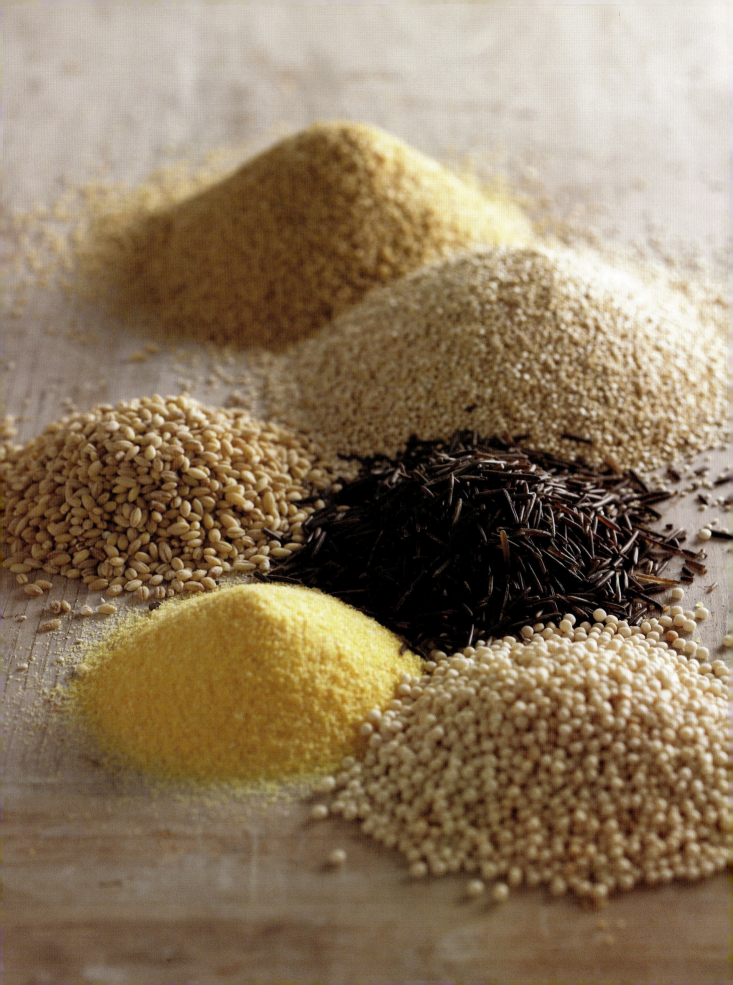

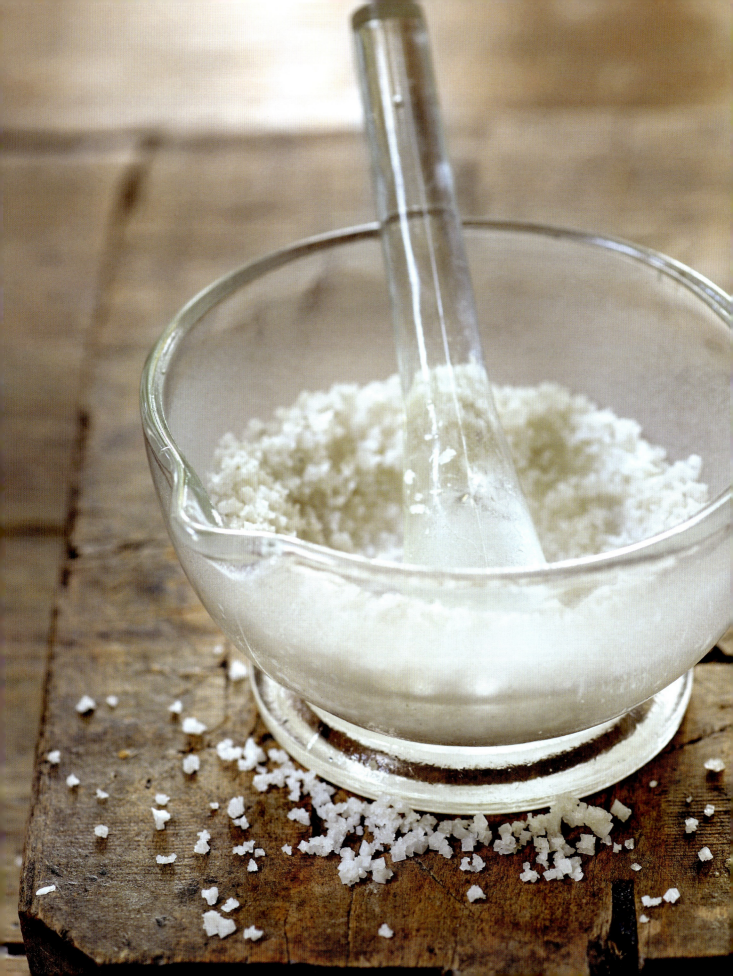

Salt

Choose a quality natural sea or rock salt that is unrefined and unprocessed and free of anticaking agents or artificial additives such as iodine. You do need iodine, but add seaweed into your diet for a natural source, or choose sea salt, which contains a natural source of iodine. Buy salt locally. Australian salts include Murray River salt, which is harvested from underground saline water in Victoria's Murray Darling River region, or hand-harvested Australian sea salt.

Salt is essential for your health. It maintains the electrolyte balance inside and outside of cells, and is important for hydration in our bodies. However, salt can be detrimental if it comes from a processed and refined source or as found in processed and packaged foods. Too much salt from these sources increases the risk of health problems, including high blood pressure, strokes and coronary heart disease.

Soy

For decades soy has been used as an ingredient in many processed foods. There is soy lecithin in chocolate, soy fibre and soy flour in breads and biscuits, and soybean oil in vegetable oils. Soy milk, soy yoghurt and soy cheese are used to replace dairy products, and soy is used as a traditional Asian food in soy sauces, tofu, tempeh and miso. The problem with soy is that when used as an alternative to allergenic foods such as dairy and gluten and as an animal protein replacement, it is consumed in quantities that are too large for your body to cope with, and it hasn't undergone the fermentation process that renders it digestible.

Soy is industrially grown, often in countries that don't even consume it, so it is produced solely for export to westernised countries. It doesn't grow naturally on a grand scale and there are environmental consequences when, for example, rainforests are cut down to grow soy plantations. Asians use soy as a well-prepared condiment, made through fermentation processes and not used to replace milk, meat or seafood. Choose traditionally fermented organic soy sauces and miso pastes. Skip the rest; they are too hard on the digestion.

Condiments

These are products created to flavour food. They have some healthy ingredients but mostly they are full of artificial flavours and monosodium glutamate, and are highly processed for preservation, such as pasteurisation or by the addition of chemical additives and refined salt. Even if these foods are organic, they are generally not healthy because the good-quality ingredients have been processed, and as a result are devoid of nutrients. Some are better than others, so be discerning. The fewer ingredients, the better. Rather than buying a premade sauce, dressing, spread or paste, make your own with quality food ingredients. Make a simple dressing of olive oil and lemon juice, natural salt and pepper. For more delicious sauces and dressings, see page 116.

Stock: cubes, liquid and powder

Stock is a flavoured water preparation and forms the basis of many dishes, particularly soups, stews, casseroles and sauces. Stock cubes, also known as bouillon cubes, are made from dehydrated vegetables, meat stock, a small portion of fat, salt and seasonings and shaped into a small cube, or the dehydrated stock is left in a powdered form. In addition to these natural ingredients they often also contain flavour enhancers, either yeast extract or monosodium glutamate.

Liquid stock is dehydrated stock, with the addition of water, which has undergone ultraheating, canning or aseptic processing to sterilise or preserve the product. Best avoid and make your own stock from scratch with quality ingredients such as pastured animal bones or non-farmed seafood, vegetables, apple cider vinegar to help break down the bones, natural salt and water. For bone stock recipes refer to page 214. You can freeze bone stock in ice cube trays or small containers to preserve for use in your next meal.

An exception is that some quality pastured butchers are boiling down bones to create quality premade stocks without any additives or refined salts. Keep an eye out for these.

Chocolate

Cocoa powder is also known as cacao powder and is extracted from the cocoa bean. Cocoa solids contain 230 milligrams of caffeine per 100 grams. Cocoa beans are fermented and dried. In a factory, the beans may be roasted. Next they are cracked and then shelled, resulting in pieces of beans called nibs. Most nibs are ground, using various methods, into a thick creamy paste, known as chocolate liquor or cocoa paste. This is then further processed into chocolate by mixing in more cocoa butter and sugar, and sometimes vanilla and an emulsifier, then it is refined and tempered. Alternatively, it can be separated into cocoa powder and cocoa butter using a hydraulic press.

Commercial chocolate preparations include soy lecithin or vegetable oils, such as sunflower oil, replacing cocoa butter, milk powder, sugar and additives. Traditional and healthier methods make chocolate from cocoa powder (not heat treated so it retains its antioxidant properties) and cocoa butter, evaporated cane sugar or coconut sugar and natural flavour such as vanilla, orange or mint.

The fundamental difference between commercial chocolate and raw chocolate is that the cocoa in raw chocolate is never heated above 45°C. This means all the natural antioxidants, enzymes and nutrients remain intact and free of processed ingredients such as the emulsifier soy lecithin. Commercial chocolate is roasted at 130°C, though this process may rid it of the vast majority of phytic acid, which is another concern with chocolate. Enjoy small quantities of this 'food of the gods' by choosing high-quality organic chocolate that is free of milk solids and emulsifiers.

Sweeteners

Sweeteners are not a food group and are best used as a spice: sparingly or not at all. The better types are those from a raw state that are produced using sustainable agricultural methods, such as honey and coconut sugar. If you use stevia, choose an organic green leaf that is naturally dried and powdered.

Ancient honey: Humans began gathering honey at least 8000 years ago. It has been used for medicinal, preservative, sweetening and religious purposes. In ancient times, people didn't eat as many carbohydrates as we do now, so were able to tolerate more honey, but this is no longer the case. Our modern diet tends to include far too many carbohydrates, leading to diabetes and obesity. Honey is two-thirds fructose and one-third glucose. Use it sparingly and buy good-quality, organic raw honey.

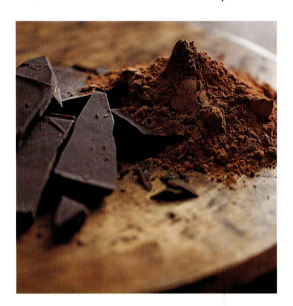

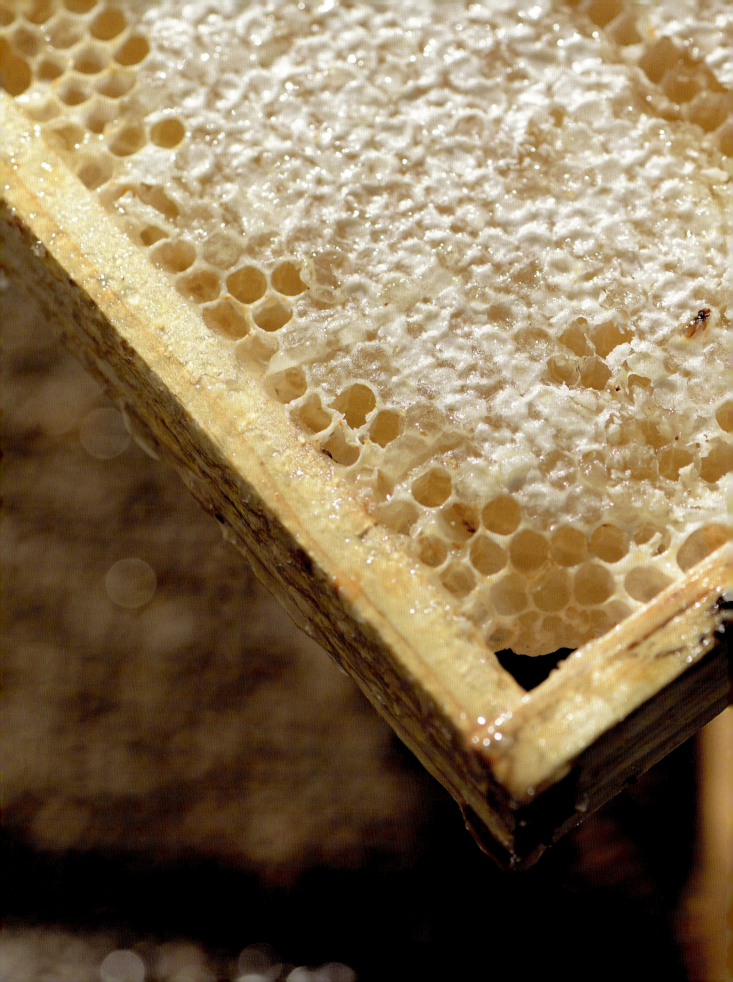

Drinks

Fluids are essential for health and the best one is water in its natural state, especially if it comes from a spring. However, bottled spring water is not necessarily ideal, as this contributes to environmental costs, from plastic bottles filling up our landfills, to the fossil fuels used to transport it, and the pollutants that the manufacture of plastics contribute to our atmosphere.

Sparkling mineral or spring water is created by dissolving carbon dioxide in mineral water. Both are fine, but always consider the source — has it travelled thousands of kilometres to get to you? Filtered tap water is less costly to our environment.

Filtered tap water is best, with a sprinkling of natural salt to every glass of water, which adds minerals similarly found in spring water and in the body. Make sure it is just enough salt to soften the water, but not enough to make it taste salty. The natural minerals aid hydration inside our cells and are fine for those with high blood pressure or kidney stones, as adding natural salt is like adding essential minerals rather than refined sodium chloride, which contributes to these conditions.

Alcohol

In European countries, a glass of wine is traditionally savoured and seen as a natural complement to a meal. In our stressed-out culture, however, alcohol has become an addictive drug, used to break down social barriers and distract and alleviate stress and emotions. Consumption is high and the consequences put a strain on our emotional and physical health. A fatty, toxic liver is a common condition caused by excessive alcohol consumption, as are gout, diabetes and obesity.

Buy high-quality organic, preservative-free wines. Enjoy one glass to complement a meal, have plenty of alcohol-free days or weeks and avoid alcohol if you have a chronic health condition.

Resveratrol is a polyphenol antioxidant, found in red wine, which has been known to reduce tumours. There is growing evidence that the health benefits of red wine are related to its non-alcoholic components. Berries are another rich source of this antioxidant.

Bitters are alcoholic beverages which are flavoured with herbal essences and have a bitter or bittersweet flavour. Numerous brands of bitters were formerly marketed as patent medicines, but are now considered to be digestifs, rather than medicines. Many European countries, as well as North and South America, have had bitters as part of their traditional cultures.

Coffee

Coffee has become an addictive beverage that is abused in Western society. It is consumed to compensate for depleted energy and to help the brain focus, and the more we drink, the more we need. Organic short or long black coffees are best. Instead of the steamed, heated milk used in cafe lattes, flat whites and cappuccinos (the high temperatures destroy the natural goodness of milk), add a dash of cold high-quality milk or cream instead. Avoid instant varieties, which are highly processed and contain additives.

Juice, cordials and soft drinks

I consider juice to be no different to cordials or soft drinks when it comes to sugar content, and all three are highly processed. Juices without preservatives are usually pasteurised to give them a long shelf life, but this destroys

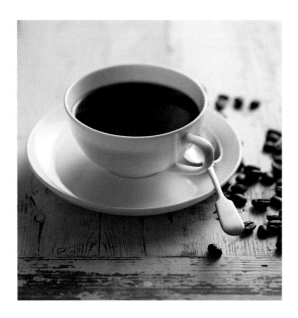

the natural nutrients. They contain too many carbohydrates; you would never eat this amount of fruit in one sitting.

Soft drinks are often caffeinated, deplete the adrenal glands and cause anxiety and high blood pressure in excessive consumption. They also include artificial sweeteners, which are known toxins and possible carcinogens. Best avoid all three as they also contribute to tooth decay, as well as the overall risk of stroke.

Naturally fermented fizzy drinks such as beet kvass and ginger ales are traditional beverages. Refer to page 222 for delicious fermented drink recipes.

Sports drinks

The idea behind a sports drink is to rehydrate with a mineral and glucose fluid during and after intense exercise. My concern is that they are usually made from highly processed ingredients and have all sorts of artificial flavours and colours added. Make a natural hydrating fluid out of herbal teas (mint, nettle, dandelion and licorice root) that have been allowed to cool. Add natural salts for electrolytes and coconut oil for energy.

Tea

Carefully select teas by looking at the ingredients on the packet. Tea often has ingredients other than the dried tea leaves, herbs or spice. Earl grey is usually synthetically flavoured, rather than having the bergamot rind essential oil added. Many herbal and green teas are also synthetically flavoured and even sweetened.

Choose local organic teas, as tea is often imported and can be irradiated when it enters Australia. Choose whole spices and larger leaves as this means more natural flavour and natural health constituents are preserved, rather then ground herbs that fill up tea bags. Ovvio Organic Teas are certified organic and are made from loose leaves, pods, seeds, bark, flowers, twigs and fruit.

Teabags themselves can also be a problem if they are bleached. Teabags are mostly made from paper, produced from a blend of wood and vegetable fibres. Both wood and vegetable pulp are usually chlorine-bleached, meaning that small amounts of toxic chlorine compounds may end up in teabag paper.

Water filters

Water filters were invented out of concern for how our tap water is being treated. Chlorine, fluoride, manganese, heavy metals, plastics and microbial pathogens such as E.coli and Cryptosporidium are either added or already present in our water and are of concern. There are many types of filtration systems that function to eliminate these unwanted toxic substances. I recommend a reverse osmosis water filter system, or if you are renting a portable counter top version with a microfilter made from ceramic and a carbon core for the best water you can get.

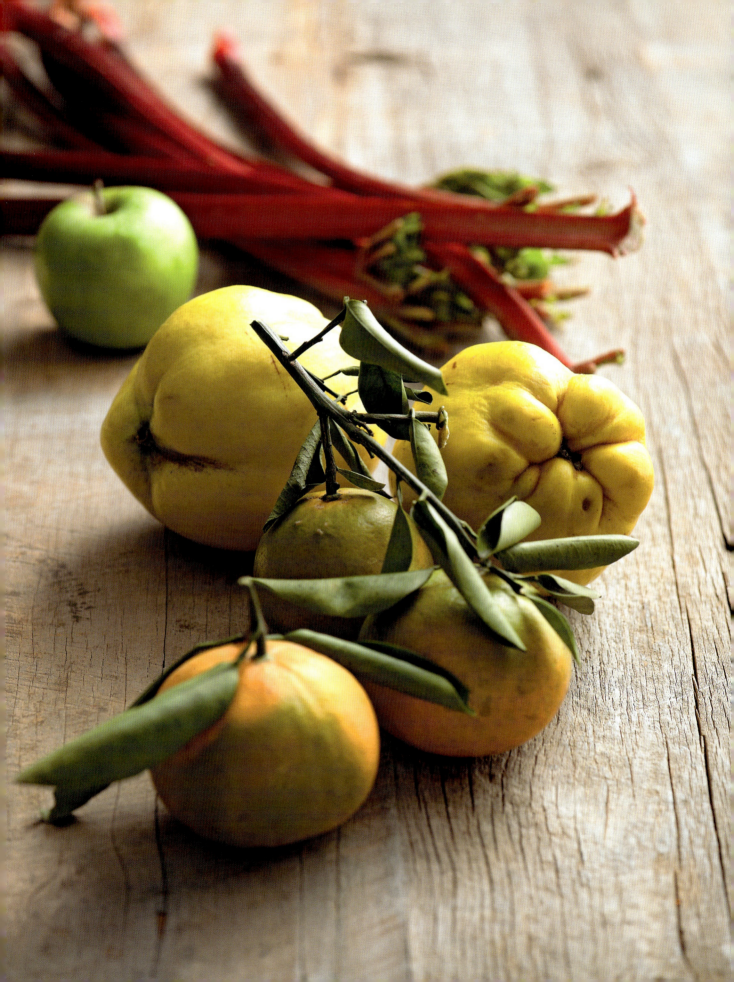

Cleansing – making the transition

This section is all about putting it together and what to eat every day to create exuberant health and prevent disease. I have outlined the considerations that affect the source of our food, processing methods to avoid and preparation methods to choose, and how to choose conscious, sustainable wholefoods and fluids. My guidelines are based on pre-industrialised food and what we have evolved to eat.

Modern hunter-gatherers
I define a modern hunter-gatherer as one who eats both animals and plants. We live in a modern society where we still need to forage, hunt and gather our food, but rather than doing this out in the wilderness, we seek out the farmers who raise animals and grow our plants as nature intended and seek out producers who take a mindful approach to their sources and preparation methods.

I call these farmers conscious, sustainable agriculturists because they are concerned with the science, art and business of cultivating healthy nutrient-dense soil, producing sustainable crops and raising healthy livestock. These farmers have the most noble profession because they provide us with the fundamental fuel for life: food.

How do you feel?
The following symptoms cry out for a change, a transition to wholefood eating and a sustainable, healthy lifestyle: extra weight, fluid retention, fatigue, dull skin and hair, itchy skin, acne, allergies, yellow or bloodshot eyes, excessive body odour, weakened immune system, bloating, indigestion, reflux, poor bowel health, brain fog, irritability, depression, hormonal imbalance, pain and inflammation and nutritional deficiencies.

The grass *is* greener on the other side!
Removing industrialised foods and changing lifestyle habits that keep us unwell or just coping can be uncomfortable. You may experience detox symptoms, a flare-up of existing symptoms, fatigue and indigestion (especially

after eating processed foods). If you rely on a lot of convenience food, changing your habits can require quite a bit of time and effort.

The transition takes time, education, healing and a desire to change and be healthy. It removes toxins and chemicals found in processed foods as well as stimulants and addictive substances, such as caffeine and sugar. It releases stored toxins and chemicals by toning and cleansing the organs of detoxification: liver, lymphatics, lungs, urinary, skin. And finally, it is a return of what we have evolved to be able to eat whilst taking a load off the digestive system. Repairing digestive function enables better breakdown, assimilation, metabolism and utilisation of nutrients – the building blocks of health. The following steps will assist you in your transition, your evolution to exuberant health!

Let's get started

1. **Take stock**

   Do a stocktake of your fridge, pantry and snack foods. Discard all processed foods with processed ingredients – whether 'natural' or chemical. (Refer to pages 22–7)

2. **Make time**

   It can be hard to find time in your day and week to plan, shop, prepare and even eat meals, but it's vital for your health. See page 58 for a simple shopping list. Try keeping a notepad on your desk at work to jot down things you need as you think of them, or use the train trip home as time to plan meals.

3. **Plan your meals for the week**

   I've given more specific details about meal planning in the Recipes section starting on page 85, but here is an overall guide, based on three meals per day, and approximate quantities. In addition, have one or two snacks each day if you use a lot of energy, for example if you exercise a lot, are going through a period of enhanced stress, or are pregnant. What suits you will depend on individual metabolism, digestive capabilities, any medications you might be taking, and body size.

EACH WEEK

3–4 cups of bone stock as a base in meals or consumed as is.

2 serves of organ meats: liver, heart, kidney or brains. (1 serve = 1 small handful).

2–3 serves of nuts and seeds (1 serve = 1 very small handful).

0–1 cup of cooked pseudocereals such as quinoa, amaranth and buckwheat.

0–1 cup of cooked beans or legumes.

0–1 serve of sprouted grain or sourdough bread.

EACH DAY

1–2 serves of meat, poultry or seafood (1 serve = 1 palm full) which includes beef, lamb, pork, chicken, duck, seafood and fish.

2 eggs (2 eggs = 1 serve of meat. Extra eggs can replace meat.)

2 serves of vegetables or salad (1 serve = 1 cup).

1–2 serves of fruit (1 serve = half a cup).

1–2 serves of cultured dairy. A serve would be 1 finger-length of cheese, 1 cup of yoghurt or 1 glass of milk (avoid if you are lactose-intolerant, and try to eat more cultured vegetables).

2–3 tablespoons plant fats, such as olive oil and coconut oil.

1–2 tablespoons of butter or ghee (avoid if you are lactose-intolerant; remember that other animal fats are found naturally in dairy, eggs and meat).

2 tablespoons of cultured vegetables (especially if you are dairy intolerant and cannot have cultured dairy)

Natural salt, apple cider vinegar, herbs and spices and seaweed to season food.

4. **Wean yourself off toxins**

Gently remove sugar, caffeine, processed grains and dairy, yeast, alcohol and over-the-counter, self-prescribed supplements from your diet. It isn't until we stop consuming these foods and drinks that we realise how addicted we are to them. They offer quick energy and distraction, a false sense of calm and satisfaction and in the case of caffeine, a laxative effect, keeping you addicted and constantly craving sweets and needing to graze.

Eliminate sugar and sources of added sugar. Instead of sugar, use sweet spices such as vanilla bean, green-leaf stevia and cinnamon. Reduce your intake of sweet fruit such as grapes and melons and develop a taste for tart or sour fruits, and the subtle sweetness present in these fruits. Reduce your intake of starchy or sweet vegetables such as peas and potatoes. These foods can keep you addicted to sugar during your transition.

Eliminate caffeine found in tea, chocolate, coffee and soft drinks. Slowly reduce coffee by half a cup every second day to avoid a caffeine withdrawal headache.

Eliminate processed grains and consume some pseudocereals such as amaranth, quinoa and buckwheat, and some wild or biodynamic rice a couple of times per week during the transition.

Eliminate processed dairy and dairy substitutes such as those based on soy, grain or nuts (for example, rice milk, almond milk and soy cheese) as they are poorly sourced and highly processed. Unless you're making your own lovingly homemade coconut or nut milk, of course! Give your digestive system a break from highly processed dairy products, choose full-fat organic, pastured dairy and make your own cheese and yoghurt. See page 218 for recipes.

Eliminate yeast and foods that encourage fungal overgrowth: alcohol, cider, yeasted breads and crackers, malt beverages, MSG (often extracted from autolysed yeast extract or from wheat), stock cubes or premade stocks, coffee substitutes that contain malt or yeast, B vitamin supplements with yeast extract and yeasted spreads.

Eliminate alcohol to give your liver and pancreas a break. Alcohol takes time and energy to detoxify at the expense of other vital bodily processes. It dehydrates us, depletes our antioxidant stores and messes with blood sugar levels. It can also promote the growth of pathogenic yeasts and bacteria.

Eliminate over-the-counter, self-prescribed supplements. 'Supplements' refer to naturally or synthetically derived vitamins and minerals, 'super foods' and processed fruit and vegetable products. Isn't it better to address the problem at its core? Face the issues with modern farming and agriculture that sees soil stripped of all minerals; re-balance bodies that are out of sync and facilitate sustainable wellbeing that transcends the need for supplements, doled out like medications. See pages 71–5 for essential vitamins and minerals, and the foods that contain them.

5. **Stop taking self-prescribed medications**

Come off the over-the-counter medications (unless they've been prescribed) and use natural alternatives. Over-the-counter medications are consumed too easily and mask an array of underlying symptoms and imbalances and, just like sugar, we can be thoroughly addicted to them. Common conditions relieved by these medications include pain, allergies, excess mucous, cold and flu, acid reflux, heartburn, constipation, sore throat, diarrhoea and cramps. Using natural or herbal alternatives take the load off your liver as you address the underlying reason for your symptoms. You may also discover some symptoms are actually relieved – you might have been living with side effects of the medications rather than an actual disease state. See professional advice for support and alternatives.

My wholefood shopping list

A general guide to help you choose the best foods when you shop.

Dairy Sheep, cow or goat yoghurt, cheese, milk, butter. Check that the product you're buying is whole, unprocessed, full fat, pastured, unhomogenised and organic, contains no milk solids, and is sugar- and additive-free.

Eggs Pastured, open range, organic.

Fruit Local, seasonal, organic, fresh. Less sugary and starchy types; choose sour and tart fruit – Granny Smith apples, berries and grapefruit, tomatoes, lemons, limes, avocado, pears, citrus, stone fruit, kiwi, papaya, apples. Fresh, desiccated, shredded and flaked coconut.

Vegetables Local, seasonal, organic, fresh. Less sugary and starchy types; choose lettuce, bitter greens (chicory, endive, rocket), common greens (spinach, silverbeet, chard and Asian greens), garlic, leeks, spring onions, shallots, onions, celery, pumpkin, broccoli, cabbage, kale, brussels sprouts, cauliflower, zucchinis, carrots, capsicum, eggplant, cucumber, asparagus, squash, sweet potato.

Fresh herbs Local, seasonal, organic, fresh. Coriander, parsley, basil, thyme, oregano, rosemary, tarragon, chives, marjoram, sage.

Seaweed Organic or chemical-free wakame, kelp, nori, dulse.

Grains Organic, whole quinoa, buckwheat, millet, amaranth, brown rice, wild rice. Sourdough or sprouted breads (wholemeal, wholegrain).

Legumes or beans Organic, whole, raw.

Oils Extra virgin, organic, cold pressed/expeller pressed coconut and olive oil.

Vinegar Organic, cultured with mother tincture apple cider vinegar.

Fats Organic, pastured ghee, cultured butter, tallow, lard, duck fat.

Seasonings Organic dried herbs and spices, natural salt (coarse and fine).

Sweeteners and sweet spices Organic green leaf stevia, cinnamon, vanilla bean, nutmeg, allspice, raw honey, coconut sugar.

Chocolate Raw, organic (without soy lecithin, milk powder and chemical additives) and cocoa powder.

Spreads and pastes Organic hulled tahini, Dijon mustard, fermented miso.

Nuts and seeds Organic, raw, unsalted, unroasted or activated. Blanched, organic almond meal.

Seafood Non-farmed, sustainably caught fish fillets, whole fish, crustaceans.

Pork Pastured (free range), organic shoulder (minced or diced), rib chop, fillet, loin chop, chump chop, leg, belly, sausage (grain and preservative free).

Beef Grass-fed and grass-finished, organic shoulder (minced or diced), rib steak, sirloin steak, rump steak, fillet steak, topside, shanks, brisket, marrow bones, sausage (grain and preservative free).

Lamb Grass-fed and grass-finished, organic shoulder, cutlet, rack of lamb, loin chop, chump chop, leg, shanks, necks, sausage (grain and preservative-free).

Deli meats Additive and grain-free, organic, pastured bacon, ham, biltong.

Chicken Pastured, organic, whole chicken, bone cuts, livers.

Duck Pastured, organic whole duck, livers.

6. **Repair and support digestive system health**
   Your body is the ultimate food processor, extractor, juicer and blender, but after a lifetime of eating a diet of processed foods high in carbohydrates, your ability to digest wholefoods and healthy fats and protein is diminished. Tone this function by eating or drinking bitters. The bitter taste of herbs and foods stimulates the excretion of digestive juices via reflexes from taste buds, gastrin and the vagus nerve. We should be able to eat animal products with ease and lightness; a healthy digestive system will perform this function effortlessly. In addition, respect the art of digesting well – it's a truly miraculous process! Chew food until liquid, eat in a relaxed state, avoid drinking with meals or sip small amounts of water to avoid diluting juices, and leave your tummy just satisfied, not full. Give it time and space to do its job. Allow hunger to rise in between meals, allowing your digestive juices to build, facilitating proper digestion and maximum absorption of nutrients. Constant grazing doesn't allow for this.

7. **Use herbal teas and food as medicine**
   When you eliminate processed ingredients and come off stimulants, you may experience symptoms ranging from a fuzzy head to headache, fatigue, digestive and immune imbalances, and feeling low, especially when coming off sugar. Relieve symptoms and support the detox process by using food and herbs as medicine. See the table on 65 for specific details.

8. **Eat with the seasons**
   We have co-evolved with the plant world, which means that the plants most readily available for us to eat in each different season also happen to be the ones that are most naturally appropriate for us to eat – for example, think energy-rich starchy root vegetables in winter and fresh, light salads in summer. Not only that, eating seasonally means you'll enjoy fruits and vegetables when they are at their peak. Following on pages 66–69 is a guide to attuning yourself to the seasons so you are in harmony with nature, inside and out.

28-day menu plan

This is an example of monthly eating plan guide. Your eating plan will vary depending on the season, the temperature of each day, what is in your fridge or pantry, the number of people you're cooking for, whether you have kids, your taste and appetite, your health status (digestion, allergies, intolerances, microbial status, medications, and genetic predisposition) and your individual daily routine. Sometimes lighter meals will be in order if you are stressed or unwell; if so, choose soups, broths, jelly, fruit and vegetables.

Tip: Whatever you cook at night, you can double it per person if you want leftovers. If you have more leftovers than you need for dinner and lunch the next day, freeze some for a quick dinner during the week. Shop and prepare what you can on weekends.

See following pages >

WEEK 1 | 28-day menu plan

MONDAY	Upon rising	Water or digestives and tonics
	Breakfast	Smoothie
	Morning tea	English breakfast, chai, green or herbal tea
	Lunch	Leftover roast duck salad
	Afternoon tea	Herbal tea and/or finger food plate or none
	Dinner	Duck soup with steamed vegetable salad and leftover duck meat or eggs
	Supper/dessert	Herbal tea
TUESDAY	Upon rising	Water or digestives and tonics
	Breakfast	Smoothie
	Morning tea	English breakfast, chai, green or herbal tea
	Lunch	Leftover soup in thermos with cheese, fruit and nuts
	Afternoon tea	Herbal tea and/or finger food plate or none
	Dinner	Pan-fried whiting with cucumber, witlof, grapefruit salad
	Supper/dessert	Herbal tea
WEDNESDAY	Upon rising	Water or digestives and tonics
	Breakfast	Yoghurt or cheese and fruit
	Morning tea	English breakfast, chai, green or herbal tea
	Lunch	Leftover whiting with leafy greens and herb salad
	Afternoon tea	Herbal tea and/or finger food plate or none
	Dinner	Beetroot and egg salad with tuna fillet in a jar
	Supper/dessert	Herbal tea
THURSDAY	Upon rising	Water or digestives and tonics
	Breakfast	Smoothie
	Morning tea	English breakfast, chai, green or herbal tea
	Lunch	Leftover beetroot salad with tuna fillet
	Afternoon tea	Herbal tea and/or finger food plate or none
	Dinner	Mexican fajita lettuce wraps with guacamole
	Supper/dessert	Herbal tea
FRIDAY	Upon rising	Water or digestives and tonics
	Breakfast	Yoghurt, cheese or pate and fruit
	Morning tea	English breakfast, chai, green or herbal tea
	Lunch	Leftover lettuce wraps
	Afternoon tea	Herbal tea and/or finger food plate or none
	Dinner	Fragrant coconut soup
	Supper/dessert	Herbal tea
SATURDAY	Upon rising	Water or digestives and tonics
	Breakfast	Vanilla and pear bircher or quinoa porridge
	Morning tea	English breakfast tea or chai or green tea or herbal tea
	Lunch	Leftover soup with eggs
	Afternoon tea	Herbal tea and/or finger food plate or none
	Dinner	Slow-cooked spicy beef and coconut pumpkin curry
	Supper/dessert	Dessert and herbal tea
SUNDAY	Upon rising	Water or digestives and tonics
	Breakfast	Baked eggs with tomato and haloumi
	Morning tea	Coffee or caffeinated tea or herbal tea
	Lunch	Leftover curry
	Afternoon tea	Herbal tea and/or finger food plate or none
	Early dinner	Roast chicken with roasted vegetables and blanched beet leaves
	Supper/dessert	Dessert and herbal tea

WEEK 2 | 28-day menu plan

MONDAY	Upon rising	Water or digestives and tonics
	Breakfast	Smoothie
	Morning tea	English breakfast, chai, green or herbal tea
	Lunch	Leftover roast chicken and leafy green and herb salad
	Afternoon tea	Herbal tea and/or finger food plate or none
	Dinner	Lentil, lemon and garlic soup with tabouli
	Supper/dessert	Herbal tea
TUESDAY	Upon rising	Water or digestives and tonics
	Breakfast	Smoothie
	Morning tea	English breakfast, chai, green or herbal tea
	Lunch	Leftover soup in thermos with some yoghurt, fruit and nuts
	Afternoon tea	Herbal tea and/or finger food plate or none
	Dinner	Pan-fried spicy prawns with cherry tomato and leafy greens and herb salad
	Supper/dessert	Herbal tea
WEDNESDAY	Upon rising	Water or digestives and tonics
	Breakfast	Yoghurt or cheese and fruit
	Morning tea	English breakfast, chai, green or herbal tea
	Lunch	Leftover prawns with leafy green and herb salad
	Afternoon tea	Herbal tea and/or finger food plate or none
	Dinner	Baked fennel sausages with eggplant and steamed broccoli
	Supper/dessert	Herbal tea
THURSDAY	Upon rising	Water or digestives and tonics
	Breakfast	Smoothie
	Morning tea	English breakfast, chai, green or herbal tea
	Lunch	Leftover sausages and broccoli
	Afternoon tea	Herbal tea and/or finger food plate or none
	Dinner	Salt and pepper chilli chicken thighs with apple, fennel and celery salad
	Supper/dessert	Herbal tea
FRIDAY	Upon rising	Water or digestives and tonics
	Breakfast	Yoghurt, cheese or pate and fruit
	Morning tea	English breakfast, chai, green or herbal tea
	Lunch	Leftover chicken thighs and salad
	Afternoon tea	Herbal tea and/or finger food plate or none
	Dinner	Pan-fried whiting with cauliflower mash and steamed green beans
	Supper/dessert	Herbal tea
SATURDAY	Upon rising	Water or digestives and tonics
	Breakfast	Vanilla and pear bircher or quinoa porridge
	Morning tea	English breakfast, chai, green or herbal tea
	Lunch	Leftover cauliflower mash, green beans with eggs
	Afternoon tea	Herbal tea and/or finger food plate or none
	Dinner	Meatballs with tomatoes with fresh curd cheese and cucumber ribbon salad
	Supper/dessert	Dessert and herbal tea
SUNDAY	Upon rising	Water or digestives and tonics
	Breakfast	Eggs with asparagus
	Morning tea	Coffee or caffeinated tea or herbal tea
	Lunch	Leftover meatballs with raw carrots and cucumber sticks
	Afternoon tea	Herbal tea and/or finger food plate or none
	Early dinner	Roast lamb or lamb shank with sweet potato mash and brussels sprouts
	Supper/dessert	Dessert and herbal tea

WEEK 3 | 28-day menu plan

MONDAY	Upon rising	Water or digestives and tonics
	Breakfast	Smoothie
	Morning tea	English breakfast tea or chai or green tea or herbal tea
	Lunch	Leftover roast lamb salad or lamb shank with leafy greens and herb salad
	Afternoon tea	Herbal tea and/or finger food plate or none
	Dinner	Soup made from leftover lamb bones with vegetables
	Supper/dessert	Herbal tea
TUESDAY	Upon rising	Water or digestives and tonics
	Breakfast	Smoothie
	Morning tea	English breakfast, chai, green or herbal tea
	Lunch	Leftover soup in thermos with cheese, fruit and nuts
	Afternoon tea	Herbal tea and/or finger food plate or none
	Dinner	Lemon capsicum and zucchini frittata with blanched asparagus and eggplant dip
	Supper/dessert	Herbal tea
WEDNESDAY	Upon rising	Water or digestives and tonics
	Breakfast	Yoghurt/cheese and fruit
	Morning tea	English breakfast, chai, green or herbal tea
	Lunch	Leftover frittata
	Afternoon tea	Herbal tea and/or finger food plate or none
	Dinner	Marinated lamb chops with minty cucumber yoghurt dip and leafy greens and herb salad
	Supper/dessert	Herbal tea
THURSDAY	Upon rising	Water or digestives and tonics
	Breakfast	Smoothie
	Morning tea	English breakfast, chai, green or herbal tea
	Lunch	Leftover lamb chops and salad
	Afternoon tea	Herbal tea and/or finger food plate or none
	Dinner	Spicy lemon butter chicken legs with blanched silverbeet and chard
	Supper/dessert	Herbal tea
FRIDAY	Upon rising	Water or digestives and tonics
	Breakfast	Yoghurt, cheese or pate and fruit
	Morning tea	English breakfast, chai, green or herbal tea
	Lunch	Leftover chicken legs and salad
	Afternoon tea	Herbal tea and/or finger food plate or none
	Dinner	Indian fish curry with minty cucumber yoghurt dip
	Supper/dessert	Herbal tea
SATURDAY	Upon rising	Water or digestives and tonics
	Breakfast	Vanilla and pear bircher or quinoa porridge
	Morning tea	English breakfast, chai, green or herbal tea
	Lunch	Leftover fish curry
	Afternoon tea	Herbal tea and/or finger food plate or none
	Dinner	Steak and sweet potato mash and tomato with fresh curd cheese and cucumber ribbon salad
	Supper/dessert	Dessert and herbal tea
SUNDAY	Upon rising	Water or digestives and tonics
	Breakfast	Blueberry omelette
	Morning tea	Coffee or caffeinated tea or herbal tea
	Lunch	Dips, vegetable sticks and cheese plate
	Afternoon tea	Herbal tea and/or finger food plate or none
	Early dinner	Slow-cooked beef ribs with cooked baby cos lettuce and quinoa
	Supper/dessert	Dessert and herbal tea

WEEK 4 | 28-day menu plan

MONDAY	Upon rising	Water or digestives and tonics
	Breakfast	Smoothie
	Morning tea	English breakfast, chai, green or herbal tea
	Lunch	Left over beef ribs and quinoa
	Afternoon tea	Herbal tea and/or finger food plate or none
	Dinner	Soup made from leftover beef rib bones and vegetables
	Supper/dessert	Herbal tea
TUESDAY	Upon rising	Water or digestives and tonics
	Breakfast	Smoothie
	Morning tea	English breakfast, chai, green or herbal tea
	Lunch	Leftover soup in thermos with cheese, fruit and nuts
	Afternoon tea	Herbal tea and/or finger food plate or none
	Dinner	Salt and pepper chilli chicken thighs with apple, fennel and celery salad
	Supper/dessert	Herbal tea
WEDNESDAY	Upon rising	Water or digestives and tonics
	Breakfast	Yoghurt or cheese and fruit
	Morning tea	English breakfast, chai, green or herbal tea
	Lunch	Leftover chicken thighs and salad
	Afternoon tea	Herbal tea and/or finger food plate or none
	Dinner	Baked fennel sausages with eggplant and steamed broccoli
	Supper/dessert	Herbal tea
THURSDAY	Upon rising	Water or digestives and tonics
	Breakfast	Smoothie
	Morning tea	English breakfast, chai, green or herbal tea
	Lunch	Leftover sausages and salad
	Afternoon tea	Herbal tea and/or finger food plate or none
	Dinner	Frittata with vegetables and green salad and velvet avocado dip
	Supper/dessert	Herbal tea
FRIDAY	Upon rising	Water or digestives and tonics
	Breakfast	Yoghurt, cheese or pate and fruit
	Morning tea	English breakfast, chai, green or herbal tea
	Lunch	Leftover frittata
	Afternoon tea	Herbal tea and/or finger food plate or none
	Dinner	Baked fish with orange butter carrots and steamed cauliflower mash
	Supper/dessert	Herbal tea
SATURDAY	Upon rising	Water or digestives and tonics
	Breakfast	Vanilla and pear bircher or quinoa porridge
	Morning tea	English breakfast, chai, green or herbal tea
	Lunch	Leftover orange butter carrots, leafy green and herb salad and cheese or dips
	Afternoon tea	Herbal tea and/or finger food plate or none
	Dinner	Carpaccio or ceviche with tabouli
	Supper/dessert	Dessert and herbal tea
SUNDAY	Upon rising	Water or digestives and tonics
	Breakfast	Scrambled eggs with steamed spinach leaves and fresh curd
	Morning tea	Coffee or caffeinated tea or herbal tea
	Lunch	Amaranth pilaf and fresh curds and cucumber slices
	Afternoon tea	Herbal tea and/or finger food plate or none
	Early dinner	Roast duck salad
	Supper/dessert	Dessert and herbal tea

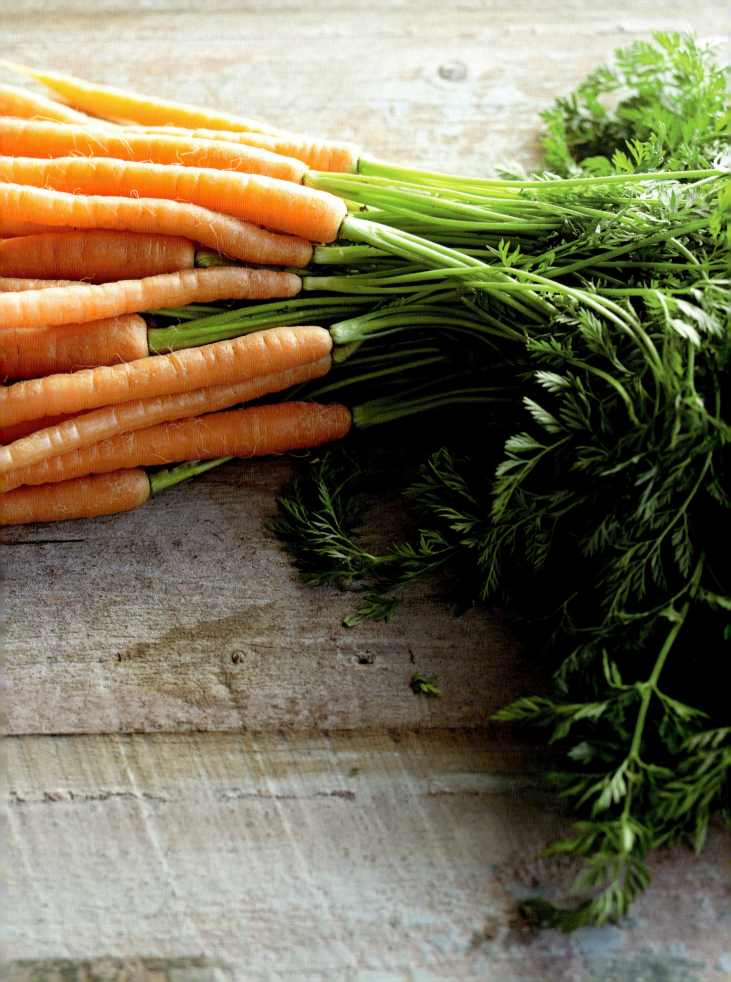

Herbal teas and food as medicine

	Ovvio herbal teas	Food as medicine
Allergies	Spring Elderflower Tea, C-Strength Citrus Tea	Papaya, kiwifruit, kakadu plum
Bacterial infection	C-Strength Citrus Tea	Garlic
Brain fog	Clarity Sage Tea and Rise & Shine Tea	Blueberries, nuts, seeds
Cold	Winter Olive Tea, C-Strength Citrus Tea	Garlic, citrus, kiwifruit, kakadu plum
Constipation	D-Tox Bitters Tea, Dandy Chai Tea Happy Bowels Tea, Derma-Kleanze Tea	Psyllium husk, slippery elm powder, olive oil, nuts and seeds, lemon juice
Diarrhoea	Silk Road Spice Tea	Slippery elm powder, probiotics
Fatigue	Rise & Shine Tea, Minty Tea, Vanilla Lemon Heaven Tea	Liver pate, coconut oil, sweet potato
General pain	C-Strength Citrus Tea, Chamomile Nights Tea	Turmeric root, ginger root
Headache	Clarity Sage Tea, Chamomile Nights Tea	Turmeric root, ginger root
Heartburn	Marshmallow Soothe Tea, Peace Bambino Tea	Slippery elm powder, yoghurt
Itchy skin	Chamomile Days Tea applied topically, Derma-Kleanze Tea internally	Aloe leaf drink (also apply externally), wild fish, olive oil (also apply externally), coconut oil (also apply externally)
Mood changes	Chamomile Days Tea Clarity Sage Tea	Wild fish, brazil nuts, kakadu plum
Nausea	Rise & Shine Tea, Ginger Root Tea	Ginger root
Parasitic infection	D-Tox Bitters Tea, Happy Bowels Tea	Garlic
Skin break-out	D-Tox Bitters Tea, Derma-Kleanze Tea	Garlic, parsley
Sore throat	Marshmallow Soothe Tea	Real jelly (made from grass-fed bovine gelatine powder)
Stress	Rise & Shine Tea, Minty Tea, Clarity Sage Tea, C-Strength Citrus Tea, Peace Bambino Tea	Bone broths, real jelly
Sugar craving	Rise & Shine Tea, Minty Tea, Paddington Tea, Vanilla Lemon Heaven Tea, Vanilla Mint Sky Tea	Coconut oil, real jelly, young coconut, cultured vegetables
General digestive support	Nourish Aromatic Tea, Dandy Chai Tea, D-Tox Bitters Tea, Peace Bambino Tea	Bitter greens, lemon juice, carrot, garlic, cucumber, cooked green apple, cultured vegetables, yoghurt
General detox support	D-Tox Bitters Tea, Pure-ify Tea, Happy Bowels Tea, Pure Flush Tea, Derma-Kleanze Tea	Garlic, carrot, celery, globe artichoke, bitter greens, psyllium husk

Spring seasonal eating

This marks the beginning of the yearly cycle, with increasing sunlight and the sense of a new start. This is a good time to make a new start or plan for the warmer weather to come. Clear past baggage and create a new rhythm for health and wellbeing. It's about new growth, new or renewed relationships and a rekindled zeal for work – the perfect time to lay a strong foundation of health. It's a time when we venture out with more energy and vitality, but it's also a period of great discomfort to many who suffer from allergies.

The following spring symptoms would benefit from a cleanse, particularly removing processed foods and drinks from the diet: • Allergies, hay fever, sinus problems, rashes, itchy and watery eyes, skin and nose • Asthma • Winter bulge and cellulite • Dry and bumpy skin hidden under winter layering

Early spring

Vegetables	Broccoli	Onion	**Fruit**	Papaya
Artichoke	Carrot	Peas	Apple	Pawpaw
Asian greens	Cauliflower	Shallot	Grapefruit	Pineapple
Asparagus	Chilli	Silverbeet	Lemon	Strawberries
Broad beans	Garlic	Spinach	Mandarin	
Beetroot	Lettuce		Orange	

Mid spring

Vegetables	Chilli	Silverbeet	**Fruit**	Orange
Artichoke	Cucumber	Spinach	Avocado	Papaya
Asian greens	Garlic	Zucchini	Banana	Passionfruit
Asparagus	Lettuce		Blueberries	Pineapple
Beans	Onion		Grapefruit	Strawberries
Beetroot	Potato		Mango	

Late spring

Vegetables	Cucumber	Potato	**Fruit**	Orange
Artichoke	Chilli	Silverbeet	Avocado	Papaya
Asian greens	Lettuce	Spinach	Banana	Pawpaw
Asparagus	Onion	Tomato	Blueberries	Passionfruit
Bean	Peas	Zucchini	Grapefruit	Pineapple

Summer seasonal eating

Nature's season of growth and maturation. We too flourish, expand outwards and mature. Summer is a time when we can connect with, and are most exposed to, the elements around us: water, salt, sand, sun and grass. Enjoy solar energy and outdoor fun balanced with adequate hydration to keep your body cool and lubricated. Thermal stress is caused by air-conditioned spaces, hot summer air and excessive sunlight. An abundance of sweet fruit is on offer. Fruit sugar or fructose in surplus can be as detrimental as refined sugar in processed packaged food, so indulge with caution.

The following summer symptoms would benefit from a cleanse, removing processed foods and drinks from the diet: • Weight gain • Bloating • Inflammation • Sluggishness • Sunburn • Hives • Sugar cravings

This is the season when we desire light, fresh and raw food – salads and raw or lightly cooked meats and seafood.

Early summer

Vegetables	Eggplant	Tomato	**Fruit**	Orange
Asparagus	Lettuce	Zucchini	Apricot	Papaya
Beans	Onion		Banana	Passionfruit
Capsicum	Peas		Berries	Pawpaw
Celery	Radish		Lychee	Peach
Cucumber			Mango	Pineapple
			Nectarine	

Mid summer

Vegetables	Lettuce	**Fruit**	Lime	Peach
Asparagus	Onion	Apricot	Lychee	Pear
Beans	Peas	Avocado	Mango	Pineapple
Capsicum	Potato	Banana	Melon	
Celery	Radish	Berries	Nectarine	
Cucumber	Tomato	Cherries	Orange	
Eggplant	Zucchini	Grapes	Passionfruit	

Late summer

Vegetables	Lettuce	**Fruit**	Nectarine
Beans	Onion	Avocado	Orange
Capsicum	Peas	Berries	Passionfruit
Celery	Radish	Fig	Peach
Chilli	Squash	Lime	Pear
Cucumber	Tomato	Lychees	Pineapple
Eggplant	Zucchini	Melons	Plum

CLEANSING – MAKING THE TRANSITION

Autumn seasonal eating

The season of harvest and the culmination of the growth of spring and summer. Autumn is the time to gather and store. Make lacto-fermented foods such as cultured vegetables and fermented drinks from surpluses of vegetables and fruit. Autumn, like spring, is the perfect time for an extended cleanse after a long period of indulgences. It is also the time to release addictive patterns to sugar, alcohol, caffeine and drugs. This is a good time to learn how to meditate, which will help overcome addictions and create awareness. It is a time to turn inwards, regroup and consolidate.

The following autumn symptoms would benefit from a cleansing of processed foods and fluids:
• Dry skin • Cracked or peeling lips • Sluggish bowels alternating with diarrhoea • Fatigue
• Bacterial and viral outbreaks

Hot spells are common during this time and while we are still eating lightly during the transition into shorter days and longer nights and cooler weather, we also eat more cooked foods. This is the time to avoid sugar and alcohol and to taste the natural sweetness of the new season's foods.

Early autumn

Vegetables	Eggplant	Witlof	**Fruit**	Oranges
Asian greens	Lettuce	Zucchini	Apple	Passionfruit
Beans	Onion		Banana	Pawpaw
Broccoli	Potato		Figs	Pear
Capsicum	Pumpkin		Kiwifruit	Pomegranate
Cucumber	Tomato		Lime	Quince

Mid autumn

Vegetables	Capsicum	Silverbeet	**Fruit**	Mandarin
Asian greens	Cauliflower	Spinach	Apple	Pear
Beans	Fennel		Avocado	Passionfruit
Broccoli	Leek		Banana	Pomegranate
Brussels sprout	Potato		Kiwifruit	Quince
Cabbage	Pumpkin		Lime	

Late autumn

Vegetables	Celery	Spinach	**Fruit**	Pear
Asian greens	Celeriac	Sweet Potato	Apple	Pomegranate
Broccoli	Fennel		Avocado	Quince
Brussels sprout	Ginger		Kiwifruit	Rhubarb
Cabbage	Leek		Lemon	
Carrot	Parsnip		Mandarin	
Cauliflower	Silverbeet		Orange	

Winter seasonal eating

The resting season, when night's darkness equals the length of the day. It's a time when we're quiet, withdrawn, sensitive and still. It's a time to contemplate, through writing and reading, and nurture yourself and your loved ones. Strengthen the immune system, warm your heart and take the chill from your bones. Early to bed and early to rise is what is in order for this season.

Winter symptoms that would benefit from cleansing, including removing processed foods and drinks:
• Seasonal affective disorder (SAD), also known as the winter blues: • Hopelessness • Sadness • Social withdrawal • Less energy and ability to concentrate • Loss of interest in work or other activities • Increased appetite with weight gain • Increased sleep • Sluggish movements • Colds and flu • Irritability

Warm foods such as stocks, soups, stews and slow-cooked meals are a wonderful winter staple.

Early winter

Vegetables			**Fruit**	
Beetroot	Celeriac	Pumpkin	Apple	Lemon
Broccoli	Celery	Silverbeet	Avocado	Mandarin
Brussels sprout	Fennel	Spinach	Banana	Orange
Cabbage	Leek	Sweet potato	Grapefruit	Passionfruit
Carrot	Onion		Kiwifruit	Pear
Cauliflower	Parsnip			Quince
	Potato			Rhubarb

Mid winter

Vegetables			**Fruit**	
Beetroot	Celeriac	Pumpkin	Apple	Mandarin
Broccoli	Celery	Silverbeet	Avocado	Orange
Brussels sprout	Fennel	Spinach	Banana	Passionfruit
Cabbage	Leek	Sweet potato	Grapefruit	Pear
Carrot	Onion	Witlof	Kiwifruit	Quince
Cauliflower	Parsnip		Lemon	Rhubarb
	Potato			Strawberries

Late winter

Vegetables			**Fruit**	
Beetroot	Celeriac	Pumpkin	Apple	Oranges
Broccoli	Celery	Silverbeet	Banana	Rhubarb
Brussels sprout	Fennel	Spinach	Grapefruit	Strawberries
Cabbage	Leek	Sweet potato	Kiwifruit	
Carrot	Onion	Witlof	Lemon	
Cauliflower	Parsnip		Mandarin	
	Potato			

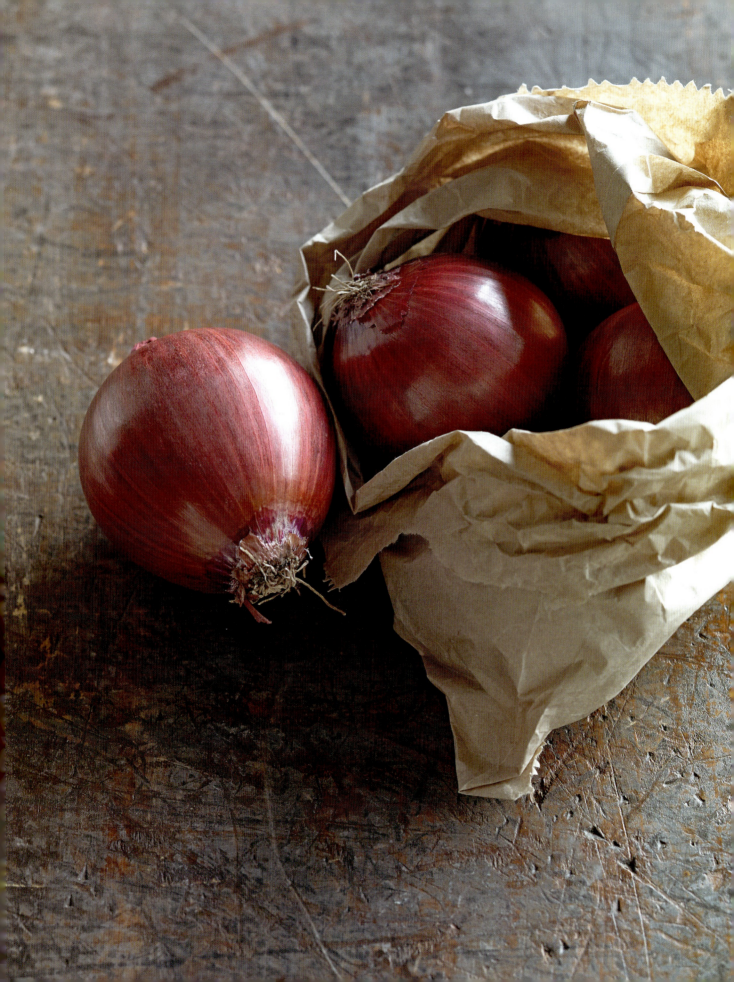

Natural sources for vitamins and minerals

Vitamin A
Acts as an antioxidant, protecting the body against pollutants and free radicals and age-related diseases and cancer. Stimulates the secretion of gastric juices needed for protein digestion, plays a vital role in building strong bones and rich blood.

Food sources: High-quality organic pastured butter, pastured egg yolk, pastured liver and organ meats, wild seafood and oily fish (sardines, herrings and anchovies).

Provitamin A/Carotene
A powerful antioxidant which converts to vitamin A in the body. The conversion is difficult to make and requires the presence of fat to make the conversion.

Food sources: Organic yellow, red, orange and dark green fruits and vegetables.

Antioxidants
These are compounds found in food which counterbalance the free radicals produced by oxidation in the body. An overload of free radicals can cause damage to the body, contributing to heart and liver disease and many cancers. Free radical production is accelerated by pollution, stress, toxins in our foods, cigarette smoking and alcohol.

Food sources:
Allium sulphur compounds – onion, garlic, chive, leek and shallot.

Anthocyanins – red, purple or blue pigments: berries, blackcurrant, cherry, eggplant peel, black rice, grape, red cabbage and violet petals.

Catechins – teas derived from the plant Camellia sinensis: white, green and black tea, raw cocoa and raw chocolate.

Cryptoxanthins – red capsicum, pumpkin, mango, orange rind, papaya, egg yolk, butter and apple.

Flavonoids – tea, green tea, citrus fruits, onion and apple.

Indoles – cruciferous vegetables: horseradish, mustard, kale, chinese broccoli, cabbage, brussels sprout, broccoli, cauliflower, bok choy, Chinese cabbage, turnip, rocket, watercress, radish, daikon, wasabi.

Lignans – sesame seeds, whole grains and vegetables.

Lutein – leafy greens like spinach.

Lycopene – tomatoes, pink grapefruit, watermelon, pink guava and papaya.

Polyphenols – thyme and oregano.

Vitamins A, C, E are also antioxidants.

B-group vitamins
All the water-soluble B vitamins work as a team to promote healthy nerves, skin, eyes, hair, liver, muscle tone and cardiovascular function; they protect us from mental disorders, depression and anxiety. Deficiency in the B vitamin complex can result in the enlargement and malfunction of almost every organ and gland in the body.

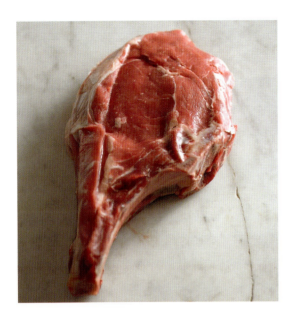

Food sources: Pastured organ meats (such as liver), pastured meat, whole grains (properly prepared), fresh fruits and vegetables (especially dark green leafy vegetables), nuts and legumes (properly prepared), wild seafood. They can also be produced by intestinal bacteria.

Vitamin C

This is found in high concentrations in immune cells, thus its potential in addressing states of immune deficiency such as colds, gum disease and poor wound healing. It is also needed for a host of other processes, which include tissue growth and repair, strength of capillary walls, lactation and adrenal gland function.

Food sources: Kakadu plum, also known as gubinge, is the richest source; fresh fruits and vegetables (particularly guava, capsicum, kiwifruit and oranges).

Vitamin D

Commonly associated with calcium and bone metabolism, including preventing osteoporosis, and it has several other functions which are equally important. Epidemiological evidence strongly suggests that maintaining adequate vitamin D levels in the blood markedly decreases the incidence of colon, breast, prostate and other cancers, and plays an important role in preventing heart disease. In fact, low vitamin D levels are associated with type I and type II diabetes mellitus. Vitamin D is important in cellular immunity and prevention of autoimmune diseases and is involved in brain metabolism; a deficiency of vitamin D has been linked to depression.

The best source is sunlight – the ultraviolet wavelength that stimulates our bodies to produce vitamin D is UV-B. Sunbathe between 10 a.m. and 2 p.m. during summer months (or winter months in southern latitudes) for 10 minutes if you are very fair and sensitive, and 15–20 minutes if you are dark. This will form adequate vitamin D before burning occurs. It takes about 24 hours for UV-B-stimulated vitamin D to show up as maximum levels of vitamin D in the blood. Because the body needs 30–60 minutes to absorb these vitamin-D-containing oils, it is best to delay showering or bathing for one hour after exposure. The skin oils in which vitamin D is produced can also be removed by chlorine in swimming pools.

Food sources: Pastured egg yolks, wild fish eggs, oily fish (sardines, herrings and anchovies), pastured lard, wild seafood and pastured organ meats.

Vitamin E

Needed for circulation, tissue repair and healing, vitamin E is a powerful antioxidant that prevents age-related disease and cancer. It is also indicated for hormonal imbalance such as PMS and infertility.

Food sources: High-quality organic pastured butter, pastured organ meats, grains, legumes, nuts and seeds (properly prepared) and dark green leafy vegetables.

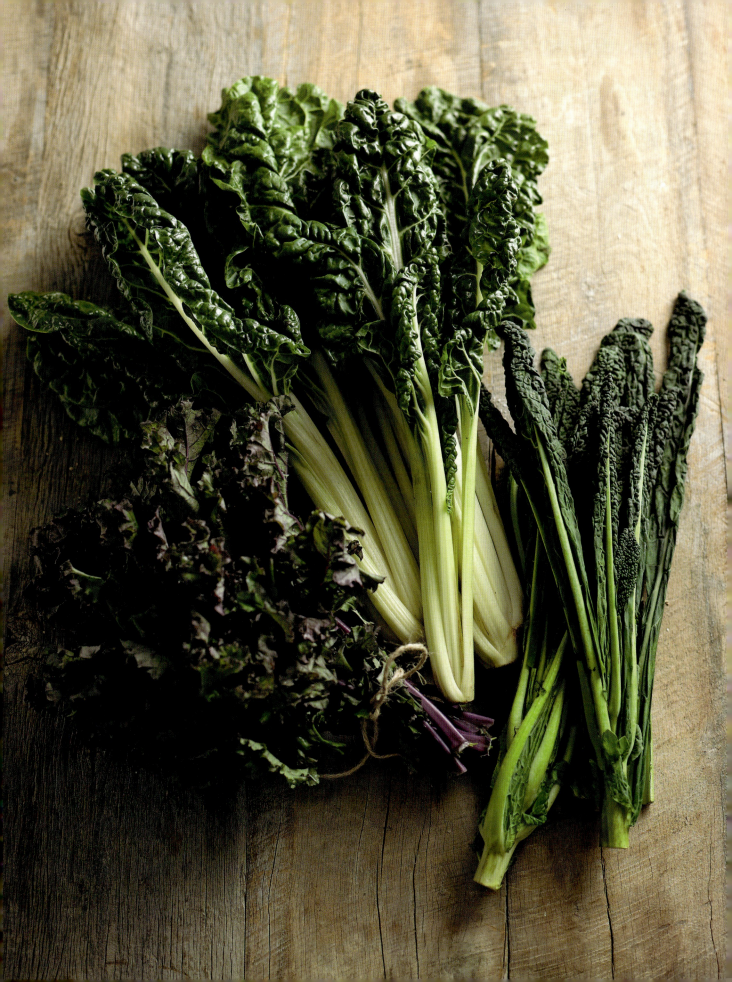

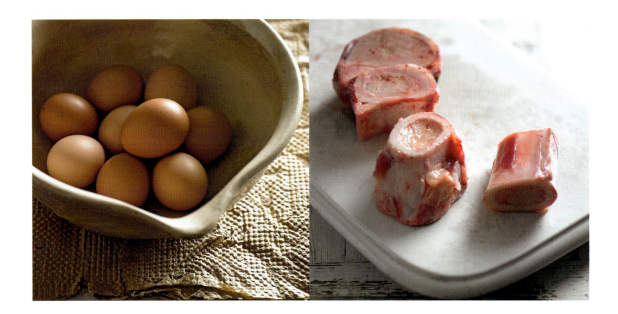

Vitamin K2
Your body uses K2 to help it channel calcium where it is needed, such as in your bones and teeth, and stop it from going to other places such as your soft tissues, where it can potentially do damage.

Food sources: Pastured hard and soft cheese, pastured egg yolk, pastured butter, pastured chicken livers, preservative-free salami, chicken breast and pastured ground beef.

Calcium
Calcium is the most abundant mineral in our bodies. Most of us know that we need it for healthy bones and teeth, but our muscles also use it to contract, our nerves need it to stay healthy, our blood uses it to regulate pH balance, enzymes need it to be active and our bodies use it to form new cells.
Calcium is best absorbed in tandem with Vitamin D. Oxalates, phytic acid and fibre all inhibit calcium absorption. See antinutrients on pages 34–35.

Food sources: Pastured dairy products (milk, yoghurt, cream, cheese); small, bone-in fish (sardines, mackerel), dark green leafy vegetables, natural salt, and bone stock from pastured bones.

Choline
Choline is essential for the health of cell membranes. Deficiencies may play a role in liver disease such as a fatty liver, heart disease and neurological disorders. Consuming greater amounts of choline during pregnancy may lower an infant's vulnerability to stress-related illnesses, such as mental health disturbances and chronic conditions, such as hypertension, later in life. Some evidence has shown it is anti-inflammatory (see References section on page 25).

Food sources: Pastured egg yolks and pastured calf liver.

Co-Q10
This occurs naturally in the body and is found in highest amounts in the mitochondria, where cellular energy is created. Levels are highest in the hardest-working tissues of the body, especially the heart. It is an antioxidant and improves the efficacy of cellular energy production.

Food sources: Pastured chicken, beef and lamb – especially livers and heart.

Iodine

The main role of iodine is to help your thyroid gland make hormones. Iodine deficiencies give rise to hypothyroidism; the symptoms include fatigue, goitre, mental slowing, depression, weight gain, low basal body temperatures, constipation, depression and headaches. An iodine deficiency can also lead to cysts in the breasts.

Food sources: organic seaweed (nori is a rich source), sea vegetables, fish and seafood, pastured butter.

NB: Certain vegetables, such as raw cabbage and kale, can block iodine absorption when eaten raw or unfermented. See antinutrients on pages 34–35.

Iron

Iron enhances oxygen distribution throughout the body, is vital for the function of the immune system and assists in the production of cellular energy. Antinutrients such as oxalates and phytates can bind to it and prevent it from being absorbed – see pages 34–35.

Food sources: pastured meat, pastured liver, pastured eggs, wild fish, green leafy vegetables. Animal sources are the richest and most easily absorbed.

Magnesium

You need magnesium for several important functions, including energy, repairing the proteins that make up your body tissue, keeping your bones and teeth strong and healthy, keeping your nervous and cardiovascular systems healthy, and removing toxins from the body. Both the brain and the heart are heavily reliant on having enough magnesium to function.

Food sources: Properly prepared legumes and nuts, green leafy vegetables, natural salt, bone stock from pastured animal bones and pastured dairy products (milk, yoghurt, cream, cheese). Antinutrients such as oxalates and phytates can bind to it – see pages 34–35.

Selenium

This vital antioxidant acts with vitamin E to protect the immune system and maintain healthy heart function. It is needed for pancreatic function and tissue elasticity and has been shown to protect against radiation and toxic minerals.

Food sources: Organic pastured butter, well-prepared brazil nuts, seafood and grains grown in selenium-rich soil.

Zinc

You need zinc particularly for healthy brain function and reproductive organs, to synthesise protein and make collagen. It also helps your body regulate blood sugar, which protects you from diabetes. It is used in over 300 enzymatic reactions in the body. Zinc has an inverse relationship with copper: when zinc goes down, copper goes up and vice versa. A water filter will reduce copper. Zinc absorption can also be blocked by high levels of phytic acid in cereal grains and legumes. You may also be zinc deficient if you have pyroluria, a condition in which kryptopyrroles, a waste product of haemoglobin synthesis, don't get excreted and build up and bind to zinc and vitamin B6.

Food sources: Pastured red meat, oysters, wild fish, nuts and seeds (properly prepared), ginger, natural salt and bone stock from pastured animal bones. Antinutrients such as oxalates and phytates can bind to zinc and prevent you from absorbing it – see pages 34–35.

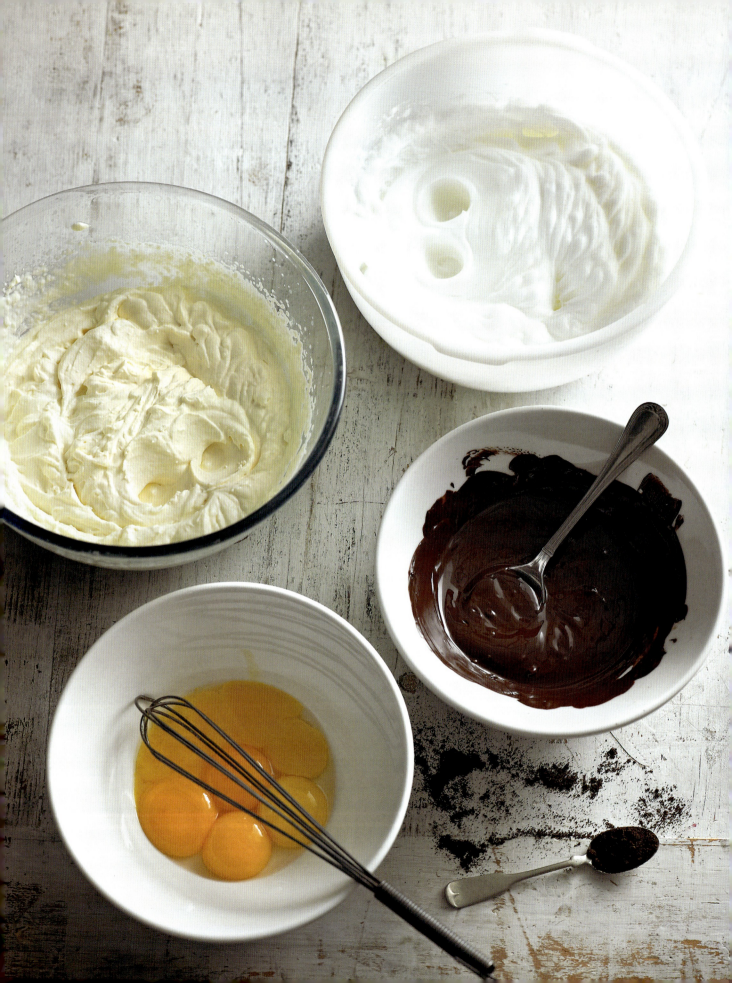

Recipes

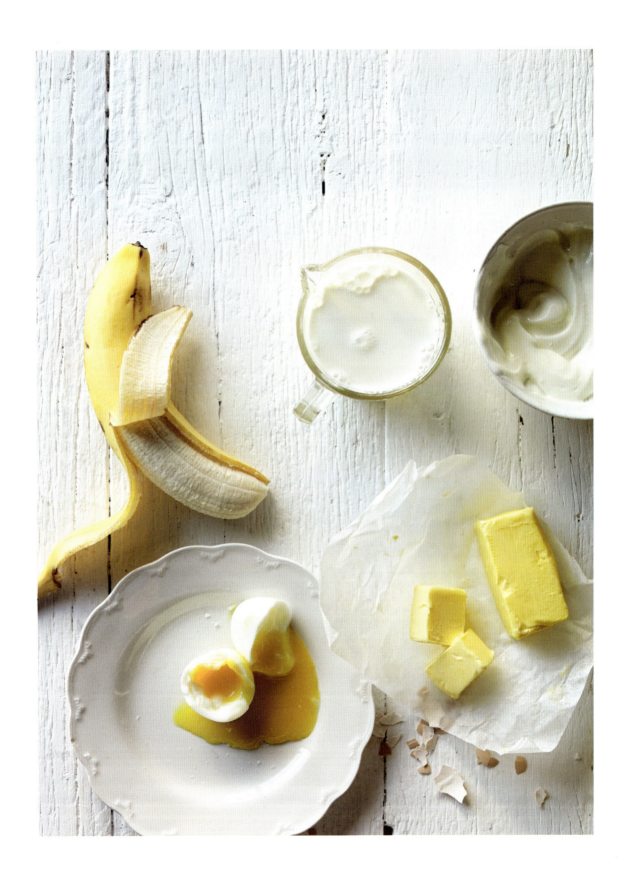

Breakfast

From the time we wake up, many of us feel exhausted, and are in a rush to get ourselves or our family ready for the day ahead. With modern industrialisation, a new way of working and living resulted in a new kind of breakfast food, offering a quick, convenient source of energy to kick start the day. This is what I call processed, nutrient-devoid carbohydrate convenience: toast with margarine, or cereal, muesli or bran with skim milk, washed down with a glass of juice and a coffee.

Even with these quick options, many people still skip breakfast or eat it in such a rushed state that they experience indigestion and bloating, and have no time to move their bowels. This leads to sluggishness and further fatigue, resulting in a day that runs by default, rather than design. And as similar days add up, disease sets in.

Create a healthy rhythm for your day from the time you wake up to the time you go to bed through making conscious choices, taking your time, and trying to be 'present'. This allows your day to flow with ease, happiness, health and exuberance.

A simple breakfast that our bodies can cope with is warmed up leftovers or a broth or soup from the night before. This is what I call a healthy, nutrient-dense convenience food.

If your palate and digestive system find this too foreign, the following recipes offer healthy convenience for familiar breakfast ideas. They are sourced and prepared well using traditional methods in order to enhance nutrition, digestion and absorption, and are easy when time is short.

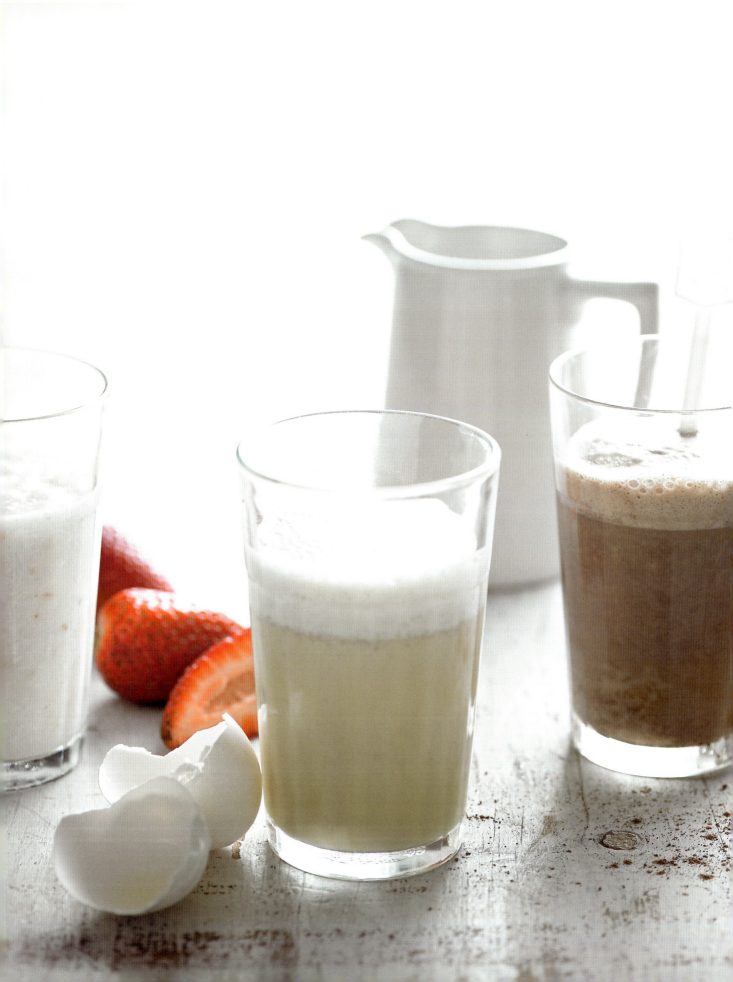

Raw whole eggs offer a complete, digestible, unprocessed and chemical-free protein source. They are the original ingredient in old-school, body-builders' protein shakes and are a fantastic addition to a smoothie (also known as an old-fashioned egg flip). Choose a base and add eggs and oil, then add your choice of natural sweetness and natural flavour.

Smoothies

Choose a base

¾ cup (185 ml) whole cow's or goat's milk

¾ cup (185 ml) whole cow's, sheep or goat's yoghurt

¾ cup (210 g) coconut milk (Open a young coconut, pour out the coconut water, then scoop out the flesh and blend together to make a coconut milk base. Store in a jug in your fridge. This is a good base if you are allergic to nuts or dairy.)

¾ cup (185 ml) almond or macadamia milk (Make your own by blending 5 activated or blanched almonds or macadamias and ½ cup (125 ml) water. This is a good base if you are allergic to dairy.)

Add nutrition

1–2 raw eggs (if you are allergic to eggs use gelatin powder from a grass-fed, healthy cow)

1–2 tablespoons extra virgin coconut oil

Choose natural sweetness

¼ teaspoon stevia green leaf powder

½ teaspoon raw honey

Choose natural flavour

1 level teaspoon raw cocoa powder (Perfect companions to this would be a drop of organic essential oil of peppermint or ½ teaspoon orange zest.)

1 teaspoon freshly grated ginger root

¼ teaspoon vanilla bean powder

½ teaspoon cinnamon powder

½ teaspoon All Things Nice Spice Blend or ground cinnamon, cloves and nutmeg, to taste

3 tablespoons frozen berries, or chopped pear or papaya, or ½ frozen banana

Smoothie on the run

Stainless steel containers with insulation can keep liquids or food hot not only but also cold. Put your stainless steel bottle in the fridge overnight. Pour in your fresh smoothie the next day and it will be kept cold until you drink it.

NOTE: The jury is still out on how many raw eggs it is healthy to consume per week. The concern is with the raw egg white, not the raw yolk. Raw egg whites are rich in avidin, a glycoprotein that bonds with biotin (a B-complex vitamin), preventing your body from absorbing the nutrient. Avidin is generally deactivated when cooked, which makes the biotin in the yolk fully available for absorption by the body. It is fine to consume raw egg yolks daily in a smoothie – simply separate the whites and reserve them for omelettes, although I believe the risk for biotin deficiency isn't as great if you are only eating a few raw whole eggs per week. See pages 71–72 for food sources of B-complex vitamins.

This most digestible dairy food offers all three macronutrients: carbohydrates, proteins and fats, with enzymes and live bacteria to cultivate a healthy digestive and immune system. Modern diets are often low in live bacteria due to over-processing. A daily source of cultured food is a good idea so if you are dairy intolerant, consume cultured vegetables for the same full-of-life bacteria and enzymes (see page 21). There are some great-quality yoghurts out there, but it's so easy to make your own at home (see page 218), so do give it a try.

All of the recipes below serve one, but can easily be increased to feed as many people as you like.

Yoghurt

Fragrant fruit yoghurt
Poach fruit with fragrant aromatic spices (see pages 234–9) and serve warm with ½ cup (140 g) yoghurt and a tablespoon or so of activated nuts (see pages 212–3).

Tropical yoghurt
Combine ½ cup (40 g) desiccated coconut, ½ cup (50 g) chopped papaya, 1 small banana, sliced, ½ teaspoon freshly grated ginger root, ¼ teaspoon vanilla bean powder and a squeeze of lime juice. Serve with ½ cup (140 g) yoghurt.

Spice yoghurt
Combine 2 tablespoons nuts and seeds, ½ cup (85 g) freshly grated apple and berries and 1 cup (280 g) yoghurt. Spice with cinnamon powder and vanilla bean powder, then soak overnight in the fridge. Enjoy for breakfast the next day.

TIP: The addition of slippery elm to your yoghurt helps feed the good bacteria in your gut and creates a soothing emulsion to heal an inflammatory digestive condition, such as an ulcer or excessive acid due to stress and a history of a poor diet. The addition of coconut oil adds flavour, satiates your appetite and stimulates fat loss.

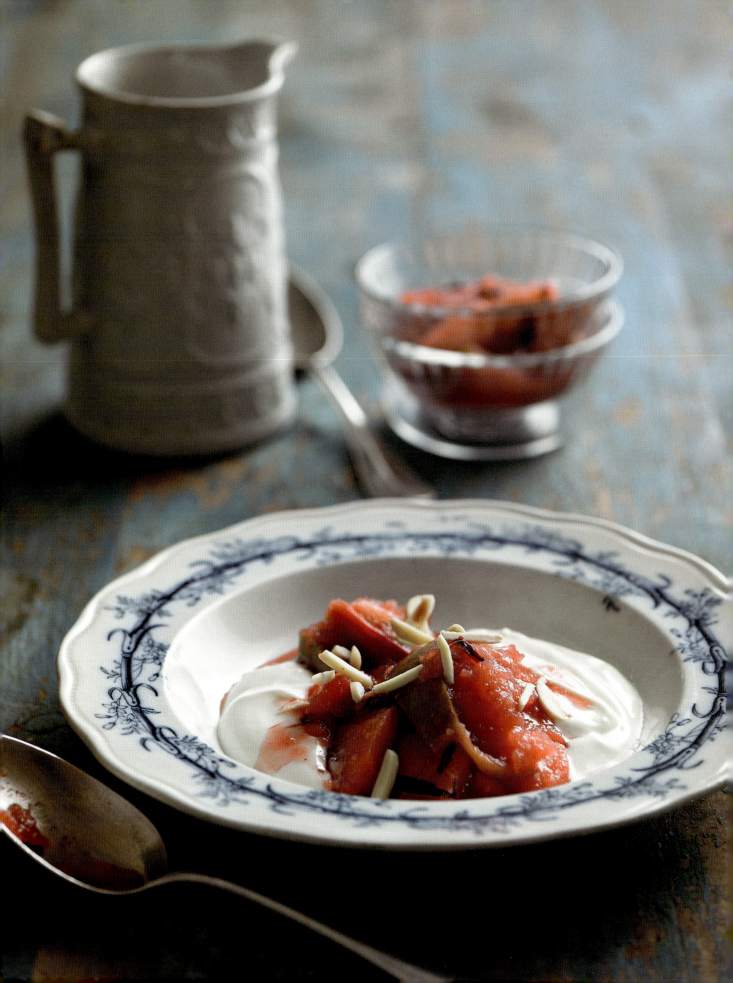

Golden eggs

Eggs are jam-packed full of important nutrients, especially the fat-soluble vitamins such as A, D and K2, and essential fatty acids such as omega-3 and essential cholesterol (healthy when it comes from healthy pastured chooks). Healthy cholesterol from healthy animals is necessary for cell membrane health in our body; brain and nerve function; assisting with learning, memory, reproductive and happy hormone production; mineral balance, blood-sugar regulation and digestion of fats through the production of bile, and is a precursor to vitamin D. The egg yolk is where most of the nutrition is found – it's so comprehensive, in fact, that it will rival any multi-vitamin.

The golden, buttery goodness of a simple egg offers the best fuel to kick start your day. Season eggs simply with natural salt and pepper or refer to the seasonings section (page 232) for more flavoursome ideas. Here are some of my favourite ways to enjoy eggs for breakfast.

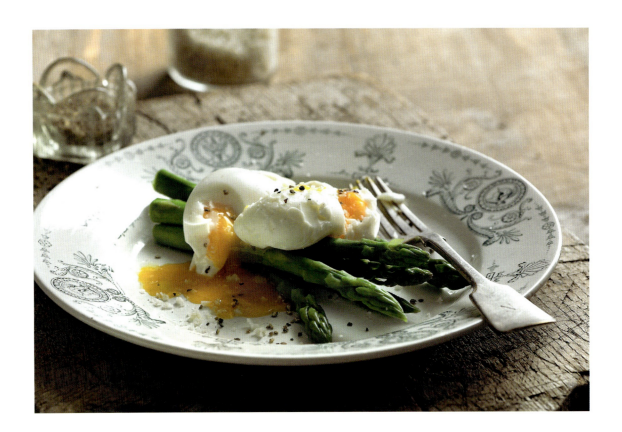

Poached eggs
served with steamed seasonal greens, dressed with olive oil or butter and lemon juice.

Hard-boiled eggs
served with chopped raw seasonal vegetable sticks or berries. Boil a dozen eggs and keep them in your fridge for the week for a quick snack or ready-to-eat breakfast.

Lightly pan-fried eggs
served with sauteed seasonal vegetables. Saute your choice of vegetables in a little butter, ghee or coconut oil. Crack 2 eggs on top of the vegetables, place the lid on the pan and switch off the heat. The eggs will cook through in the residual heat – give them about 5–7 minutes.

Omelette or scrambled eggs
with leftover vegetables. Use an adequate amount (about 2 tablespoons) of butter, ghee or coconut oil so your egg mixture doesn't stick to the base of the pan. Or make a frittata with leftover vegetables (see page 134).

Soft-boiled eggs
served on a bed of green leaves or asparagus, cherry tomatoes and avocado. Or place your egg in your favourite egg cup, crack the top and dip in steamed asparagus or toasty soldiers.

Baked eggs
in tomatoes. This is a breakfast idea that needs a little extra time to prepare and cook but is worth every delicious mouthful. See page 153 for the recipe.

Sweet berry omelette
Beat 3 eggs per person and add $\frac{1}{4}$ teaspoon each of cinnamon powder, vanilla bean powder and stevia green leaf powder. Heat a little coconut oil in a medium frying pan over medium heat. Pour the egg mixture into the pan and swirl to coat the base. Cover with the lid until the eggs form a flat omelette, about 5 minutes. Add a small handful of berries to half the omelette and flip the other half over the top. Enjoy your light, fluffy and naturally sweet omelette straight away.

For an alternative sweet omelette, replace the berries with mashed or sliced banana.

This is a simple assembly of beautiful ingredients on a plate that can be eaten with your fingers or a fork. Finger food plates make an easy meal idea for any time of the day because they take so little time to prepare. Assemble fresh or raw foods, leftovers from the night before, dips (see page 98), nuts, cheese and cultured vegetables (see page 221). Always include an animal protein and fat to sustain your energy levels until your next meal. The suggestions offered here could also be served as canapes at your next soiree.

Finger food plate

Your healthy options

Fresh curd (see page 216), tomato and cucumber slices and cultured vegetables (see page 221), with a drizzle of olive oil.

Leftover chicken meat, green apple slices and Quark cheese sprinkled with cinnamon, with a drizzle of coconut oil.

Strawberries, sliced boiled eggs, carrot sticks and avocado dip (see page 99).

Meatballs (see page 164), cultured vegetables and cherry tomatoes.

Grapefruit segments, activated nuts, egg slices and cucumber.

Homemade flaked tuna (see page 122), cucumber, tomato and avocado, with a drizzle of olive oil.

Pate (see page 228) spread on sturdy vegetables, such as celery and carrot.

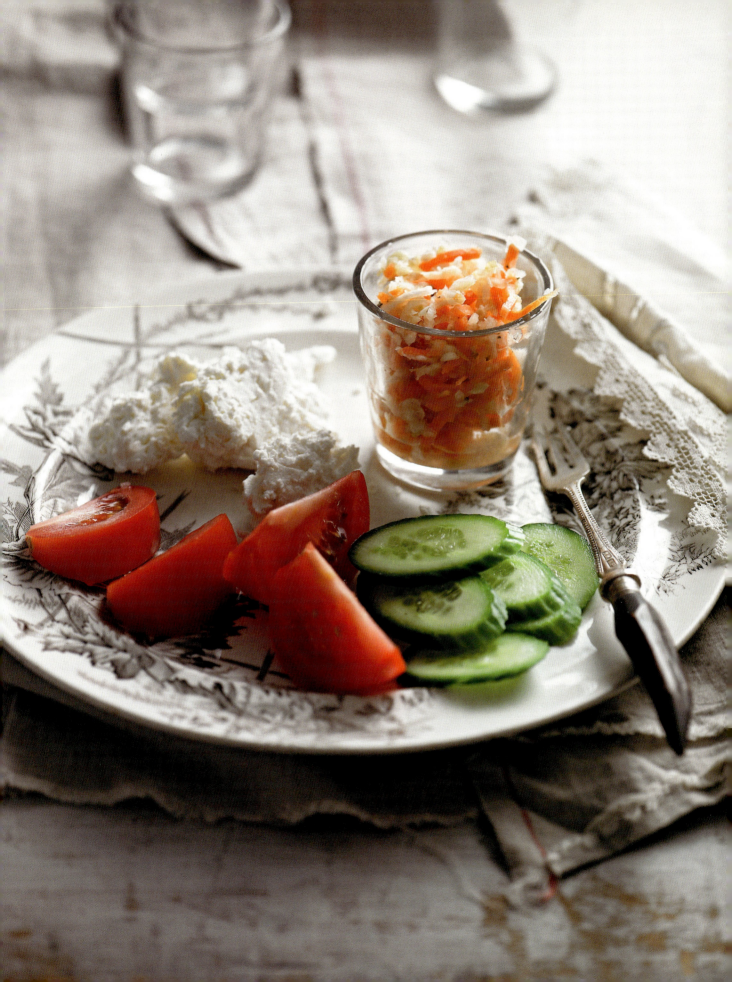

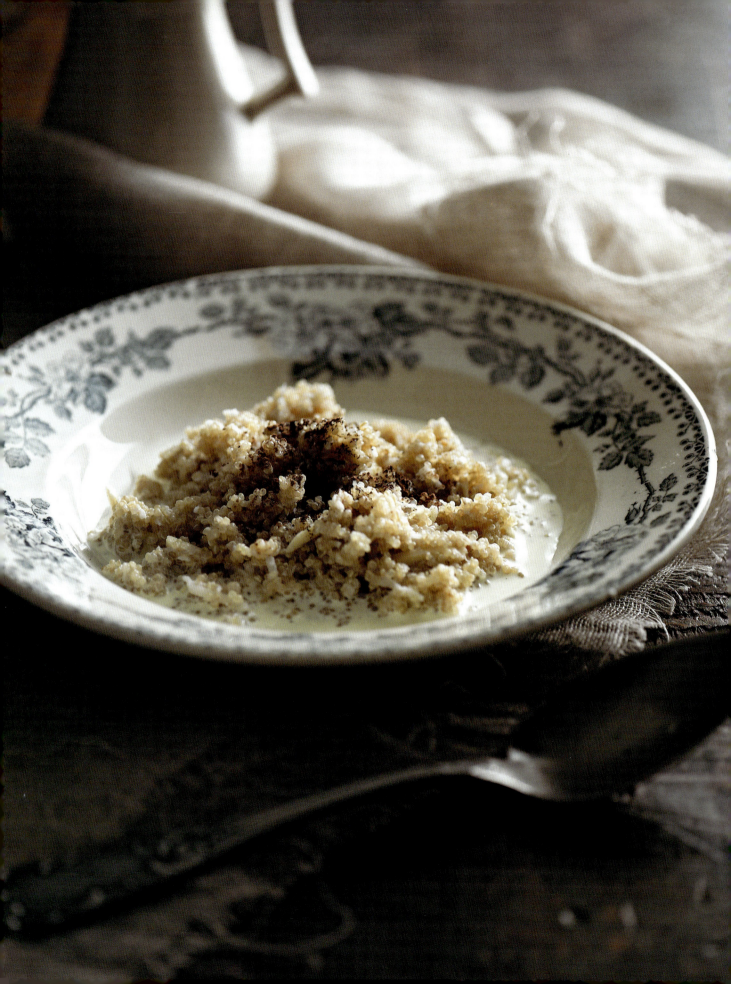

Quinoa, buckwheat and amaranth are not real grains; they are known as pseudocereals and are not part of the wheat or grass family. They are gluten free and generally easier to digest. Make a wholesome porridge by preparing these non-grains well, to further enhance digestion and nutrition, and speed up the cooking time. See page 212 (basics) for further information on soaking grains.

Gluten-free porridge

Serves 1–2 **PREP TIME:** *10 minutes, plus overnight soaking* **COOKING TIME:** *10 minutes*

1. Start by soaking the pseudocereals in a bowl overnight. For every ½ cup (50 g) quinoa, buckwheat or amaranth you will need 2 cups (500 ml) water. You will then need to add a pinch of natural salt and an acid medium. Choose one of the following:

3 tablespoons lemon juice

2 tablespoons whey (see page 216)

1 tablespoon apple cider vinegar

1 tablespoon yoghurt (see page 218)

2. The next day, drain the pseudocereals and place in a saucepan. Pour in enough water to cover (or milk if you prefer a creamier consistency) and cook through gently over medium heat. Keep adding more liquid as needed until the pseudocereals are soft and cooked through – this should take about 10 minutes.

3. Serve warm with your choice of cream, milk or yoghurt and freshly grated green apple or berries, nuts and seeds. If serving with nuts and seeds, you may like to soak them overnight with your pseudocereals.

4. Flavour with natural vanilla bean powder or cinnamon powder, sweeten with stevia green leaf powder and add a tablespoon of coconut oil for a quality fat.

Grain free, easy to digest and supportive for a sluggish bowel, this breakfast is a wonderful alternative to gluten-based muesli. It can also be enjoyed as a delicious dessert, much like a pudding.

Pear and vanilla bircher

Serves 4–6 **PREP TIME:** *10 minutes, plus overnight soaking*

½ teaspoon vanilla bean powder
1 pear, grated with skin
3 tablespoons extra virgin coconut oil
2 cups (560 g) homemade (see page 218) or good-quality store-bought yoghurt
1 tablespoon raw honey (optional)
½ cup (40 g) desiccated coconut
3 tablespoons raw almonds
3 tablespoons raw macadamias
3 tablespoons sesame seeds
3 tablespoons chia seeds
a pinch of natural salt
½ teaspoon cinnamon powder

1. Combine the vanilla, pear, coconut oil, yoghurt and honey (if using) in a medium bowl. Add the remaining ingredients and mix well to combine. Leave to soak overnight, then enjoy for breakfast the next morning.

TIPS: You can double or quadruple this mixture and store it in a jar in the fridge for up to 3 days. This is also delicious made with grated apple or ½ cup of grated or mashed seasonal fruit.

Traditional bircher muesli
To make one serve, mix together 2 tablespoons rolled oats and 3–4 tablespoons water in a small bowl, then stir in 1 tablespoon lemon juice, 1 tablespoon cream and 1 large green apple, finely grated. Leave to soak overnight.

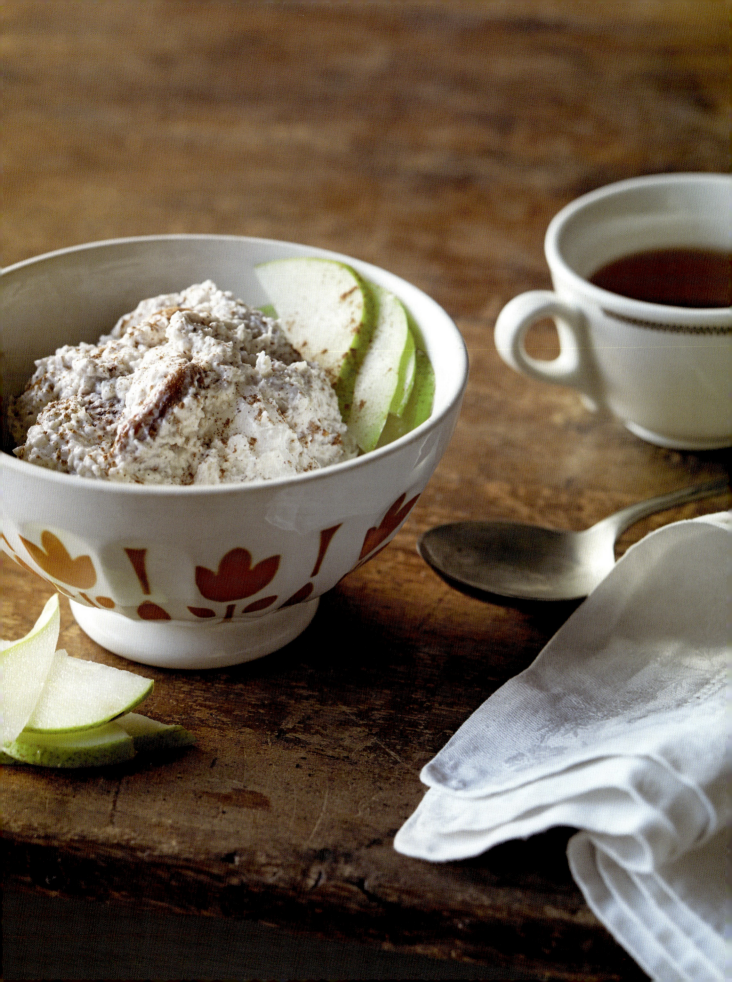

Breakfast beverages

A breakfast beverage is one to be consumed upon rising to aid digestion and stimulate a healthy bowel motion.

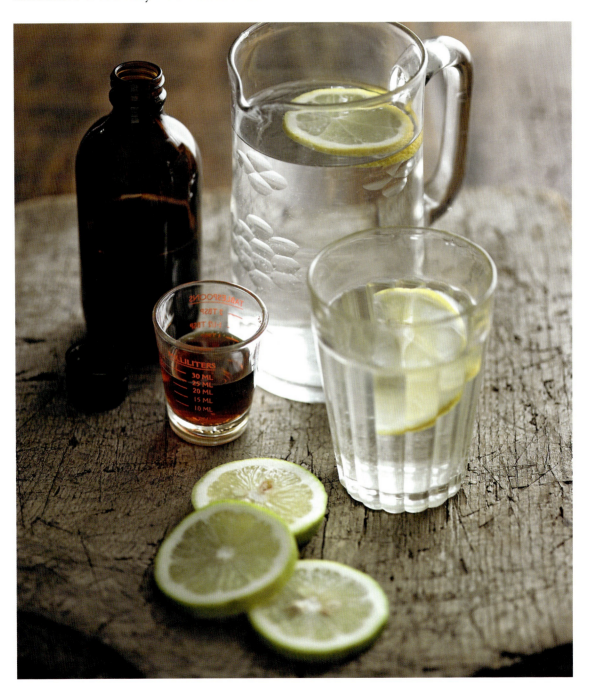

Bitter herbal tonics

These are the strongest digestive aids and are individually prescribed by your herbalist. They don't taste very nice but will help ease wind, discomfort and bloating.

Herbal teas

These are useful to sip during a meal to aid digestion. Warming teas include those made with ginger root, cinnamon bark, cardamom, clove, dill, aniseed, chamomile and fennel seed. Bitter teas are those made with chicory and dandelion root. Nourish Aromatic Tea, Peace Bambino Tea or Dandy Chai Tea (see page 232) are perfectly blended for therapeutic benefits, as well as tasting so good. Avoid caffeinated teas or drinks with breakfast as they inhibit the absorption of vitamins and minerals due to their rich tannins.

Broths

Homemade broths (see page 124) offer rich electrolytes, gelatin and cartilage. They are just the thing for healing inflammatory digestive disorders, musculoskeletal inflammatory disorders and poor digestive processes, or for those who can't stomach breakfast because of a long habit of not eating or eating on the run.

For a simple and easy way to make a cup of broth, freeze bone stock (see page 214) in stainless steel ice cube trays. Pop 2 frozen ice cubes of bone stock in a mug of boiling water. Add finely chopped fresh herbs and seaweed. If you like, add some sharpness with lemon or lime juice and some heat with grated ginger root or chilli flakes.

Fermented drinks

Kombucha or beet kvass (see page 223) offer healthy bacteria, especially if you are not consuming any cultured dairy or vegetables with your breakfast. Taking a dairy-free pure probiotic in water upon rising adds good bacteria to your digestive system if you are not used to taking fermented beverages. A quality probiotic may be obtained from your pharmacist, naturopath or health food store.

Lemon, lime or grapefruit

Squeeze half a citrus fruit and add the juice to a glass of warm water with a sprinkling of natural salt. Caution: grapefruit juice does not interact well with many medications so check with your doctor first if you are concerned.

Apple cider vinegar

Rich in enzymes and potassium, a tablespoon of apple cider vinegar stirred into a glass of warm water supports a healthy immune system, helps control weight, promotes digestion and pH balance, soothes dry throats and removes toxins.

Juice

Enjoy an easily digestible juice when your bowel feels congested or your digestion is compromised. A blend of celery, cucumber, ginger root, parsley or coriander, lemon rind and a splash of fermented drink or apple cider vinegar is just the thing. Return the pulp to the juice and give it a good stir before you drink it. The addition of a fat balances blood sugar levels and aids nutrient assimilation. Try coconut oil, melted butter or ghee.

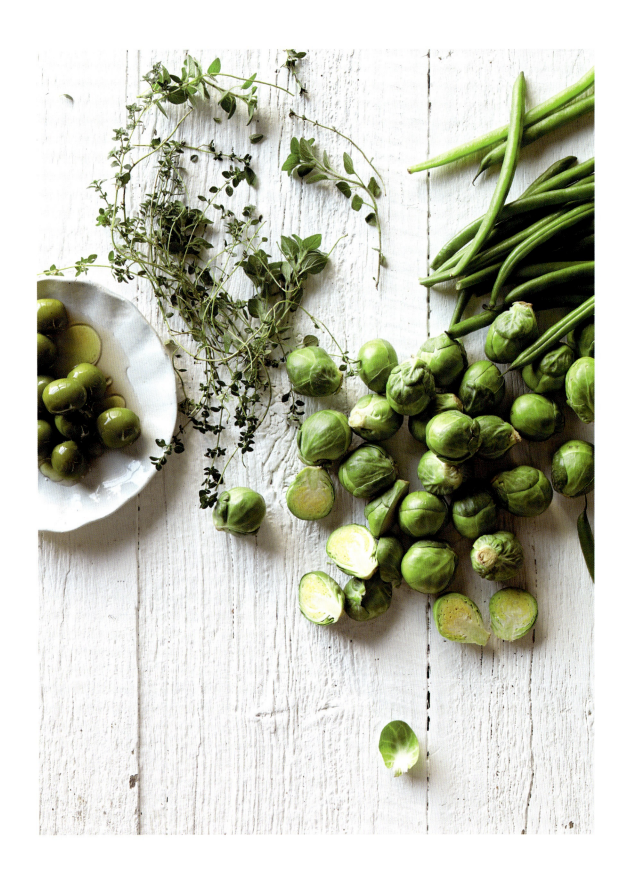

Light meals and sides

A light meal of salads and other deliciously prepared vegetables is quick and easy to create without compromising on flavour and nutrients. I call them my 'one-pot wonders'. They not only save in time and energy but also on washing the dishes. A sensible solution when cooking for one!

Light meals are also light on digestion and ideal when you're out and about. They are usually portable and easy to eat. Enjoy them for brunch, lunch, morning or afternoon tea, supper or as a snack, or serve them as side dishes. Alternatively, offer a handful of your favourite dishes as a delectable banquet spread at your next dinner party.

This idea is similar to the breakfast finger food plate on page 86 but it is assembled in a lunch box made from stainless steel or a glass container with a plastic lid. Keep an ice pack with your lunch box to maintain freshness.

Finger food lunch box

Vegetable sticks, such as cucumber, capsicum (pepper), celery, carrot and zucchini (courgette).

Cherry tomatoes.

Boiled eggs in their shells (boil a dozen eggs and refrigerate in readiness for the week ahead).

Cheese: either hard cheese cut into slices or a soft cheese, like a curd or crumbly feta, put in a small container.

Your choice of dressings and/or dips (see pages 116 and 98), stored in a small container in your lunch box.

Seasonal fruit. Keep small fruit whole, or peel and slice larger fruit (rub lemon over cut apple and pear to prevent browning).

Leftover sausages or meatballs (see page 164), chopped if liked.

Activated nuts and seeds.

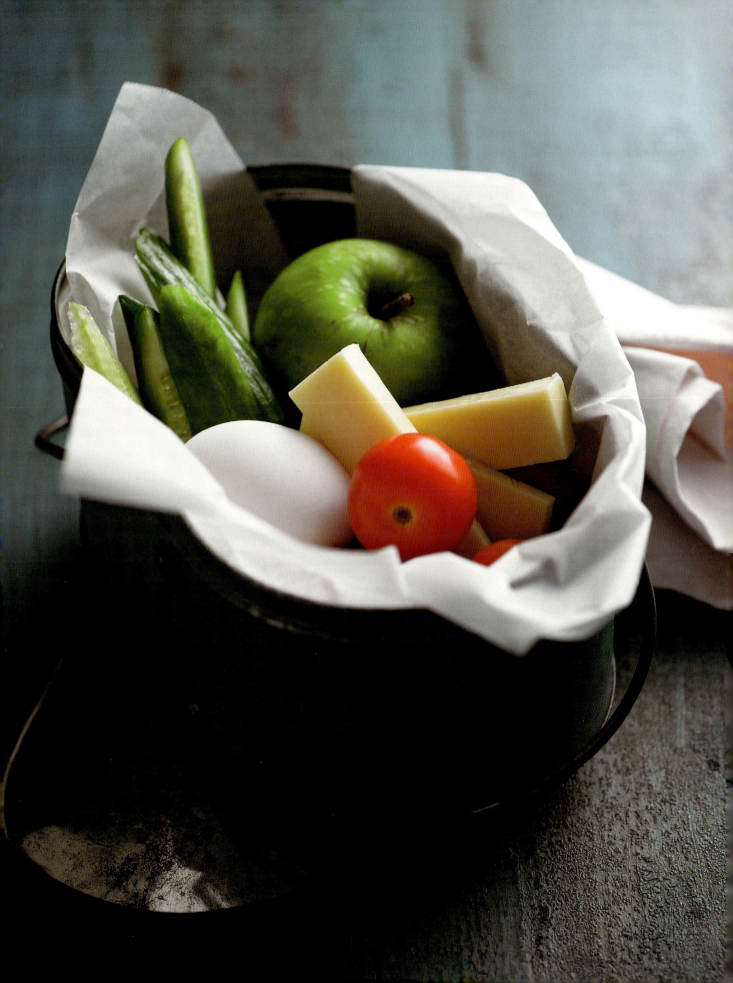

Dips

All the dips serve 4, but it really depends how hungry you are!

Homemade dips are a wonderful solution when you need something quick and light to eat. Raw or lightly steamed vegetables love a skinny dip! Choose raw vegetables that cut into perfect sticks for dipping: celery, cucumber, carrot, capsicum (pepper), fennel and zucchini (courgette) or sturdy lettuce leaves such as cos or witlof. Asparagus spears and broccoli and cauliflower florets can also be dipped but are best steamed for easy digestion. These dips will keep in the fridge for up to 5 days. They can also be served as salad dressings by adding more oil and water, then whisking into a liquid emulsion.

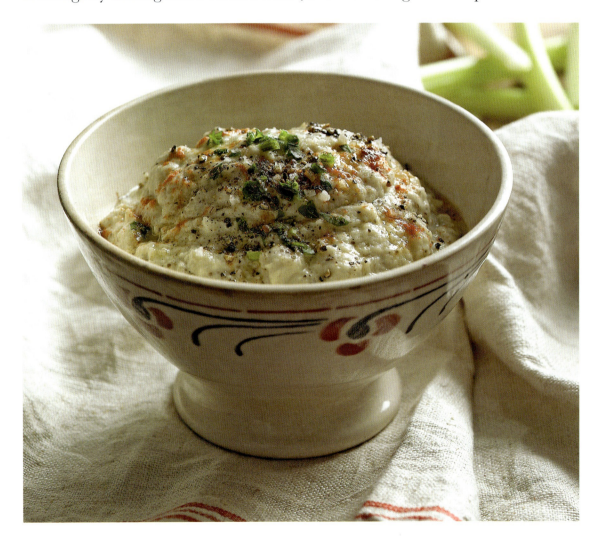

Blackened eggplant dip

An ode to Lebanese home cooking, serve this dip with Tabouli sans grain on page 118 as a delicious accompaniment to meat.

2 eggplants (aubergines)
3 cloves garlic, unpeeled
3 tablespoon fresh lemon juice
2 tablespoons olive oil, plus extra to serve
2 tablespoons hulled tahini
natural salt and freshly cracked pepper
3 tablespoons finely chopped flat-leaf parsley
paprika, to garnish

1. Preheat the oven to 200°C (fan-forced).

2. Clean and prick the eggplants with a fork. Place in a roasting tin with the garlic cloves and roast for 20 minutes or until the skin has blackened and the eggplants have collapsed. Leave until cool enough to handle, then cut the eggplants in half and scoop out the flesh. Discard the skin. Pop the garlic out of its skin.

3. Place the eggplant flesh in a food processor and add the lemon juice, olive oil, tahini and garlic. Season with salt and pepper and blend until smooth. Sprinkle over the parsley and paprika and serve with a final drizzle of olive oil.

Minty cucumber yoghurt dip

Mint, yoghurt and cucumber are cooling ingredients that will soothe an inflamed tummy.

1 Lebanese cucumber
1 teaspoon finely chopped mint or
    ½ teaspoon dried mint
1 cup (280 g) yoghurt (see page 218)
2 tablespoons olive oil
½ teaspoon finely grated lemon zest
3 tablespoons fresh lemon juice
natural salt and freshly cracked pepper

1. Peel the cucumber and grate it into a bowl, then squeeze out as much liquid as you can. Stir in the mint, yoghurt, olive oil, lemon zest and lemon juice and season with salt and pepper.

Green tahini dip

Tahini made from hulled seeds means, as you would expect, that the hulls have been removed. Even though there is more calcium in unhulled tahini, the hulled version is better as the hulls contain oxalic acid, phytates and enzyme inhibitors, all of which are antinutrients (see pages 34–35).

½ cup (140 g) hulled tahini
3 tablespoons fresh lemon juice
3 tablespoons olive oil
1 spring onion, trimmed and roughly chopped
small handful of coriander or flat-leaf
    parsley stalks
natural salt and freshly cracked pepper

1. Place all the ingredients and ½ cup (125 ml) water in a food processor and blend until smooth. Taste and adjust the seasoning if necessary.

Velvety lime avocado dip

To make a chunky spiced guacamole, mash the ingredients with a fork instead of processing them, then stir in 1 finely diced firm tomato, 1 small finely diced red onion and 1 teaspoon Mexican Herb & Spice Blend or sweet paprika and cayenne pepper, to taste.

2 avocados, peeled and stones removed
1 clove garlic, crushed
½ teaspoon lime zest
juice of ½ lime
3 tablespoons olive oil
natural salt and freshly cracked pepper

1. Place avocado flesh, garlic, lime zest, lime juice and olive oil in a food processor and blend until silky smooth. Season to taste.

LIGHT MEALS AND SIDES

Leftovers

Warm Leftovers

Any leftovers may be packed into a container and enjoyed for lunch the next day. But how do you serve them warm without using a microwave?

The answer is a thermos or insulated container. This works particularly well for stews, casseroles and soups.

In the morning, heat your leftovers on the stove top and transfer to the container while still hot. It should stay nice and warm until lunch time.

Choose a wide-mouth insulating container for stews and casseroles as you will need to fit in a fork or spoon. A small-mouth container is better for soups and broths.

For more information on the ill effects of microwaving, see pages 31–32.

Leftover Roast Salad

This is the simplest meal to make for a light meal – leftovers converted into a salad! Slice or pull apart leftover roast duck, pork, chicken or lamb (see pages 159, 169, 178 and 181) and combine with your choice of salad ingredients, such as fresh herbs, lettuce leaves, cherry tomatoes, sliced cucumber and grated carrot. Toss with a delicious dressing (see page 117). You can also use leftover cooked vegetables instead of salad leaves.

Save any congealed fat, gelatin, bones, skin, gravy juices, leftover vegetables and meat from the roast to make a stock (see page 214).

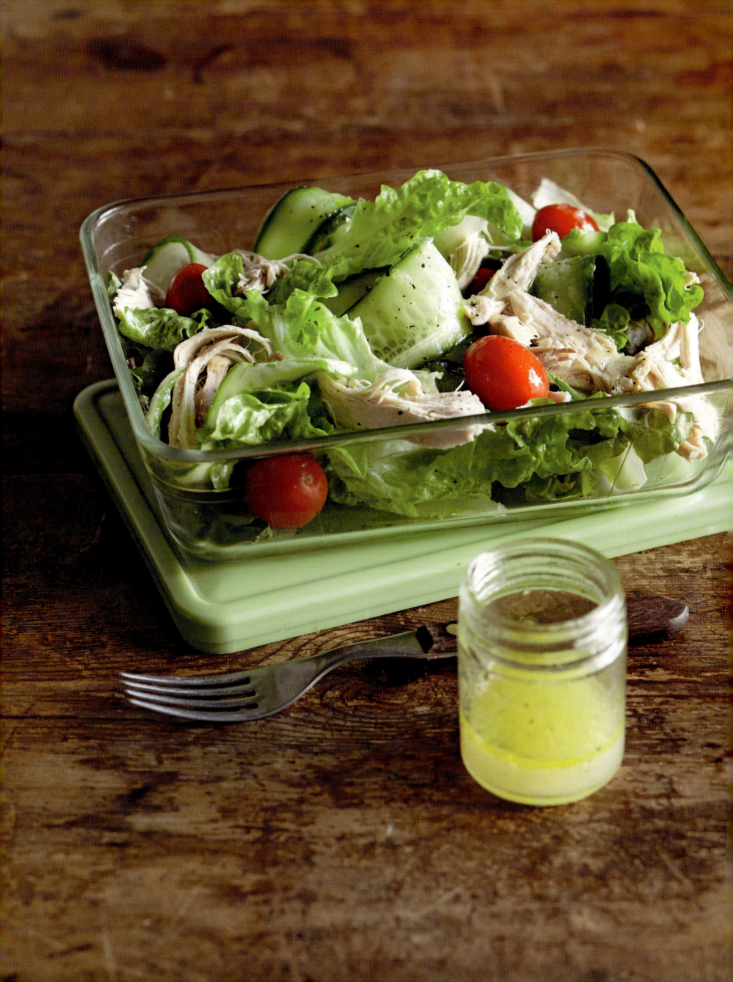

Cooking your greens

I ate a lot of greens when I was growing up. They are a staple of the Mediterranean diet – we call them 'horta', which means wild mountain greens or weeds, and like most Mediterranean households we grew them in our back yard. As a child, I loved collecting a mixture of wild spinach, fennel tops, beet leaves, spinach, nettles and rocket. My mum and grandmother would simply blanch them in water and serve them with lashings of olive oil and lemon juice. Greens are cleansing, rich in vitamins, minerals, antioxidants and bitter constituents (such as those found in artichokes), which stimulate digestive juices.

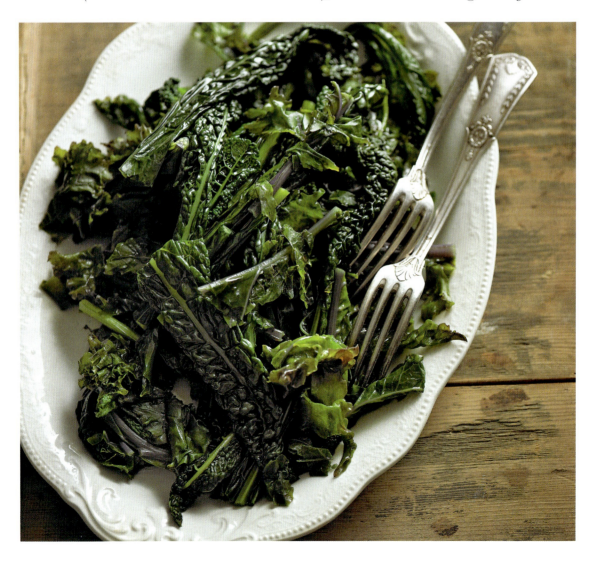

Artichokes

Trim the stem and discard the tough outer leaves to reveal the most tender leaves. Remove the tips by cutting a little above its maximum circumference, then scoop out the fluffy choke with a teaspoon. Cut in half and place in a bowl of water with a squeeze of lemon juice (this will prevent the artichoke from browning). When ready to cook, boil in salted water for 15–20 minutes. Serve with lemon juice, olive oil, natural salt and freshly cracked pepper.

Bok choy or Chinese broccoli

Saute in coconut oil, lime juice, ginger and coriander leaves and serve just as is, add it to soups or serve it as a side dish with fish or chicken.

Broccoli

Make a green mash by steaming or boiling the broccoli, then pureeing with butter, natural salt and freshly cracked pepper. Add some steamed cauliflower and cream cheese if you prefer a creamier mash. Steam broccoli florets, then grill with lots of grated cheese on top, or saute in butter and serve with pan-fried eggs.

Brussels sprouts

Steam thinly sliced sprouts, or cut them in half and boil them, then saute in butter and bacon bits and season to taste.

Green asparagus

Saute in coconut oil with finely sliced chilli, lime juice, natural salt and freshly cracked pepper. Saute in butter and bacon bits and season to taste, or simply steam until just tender but still a bit crunchy. Dip the steamed spears into soft-boiled eggs or a delicious dip (see page 98) or mayonnaise (see page 224).

Green beans

Boil or steam and toss in an olive oil and lemon juice dressing (see page 117) or finely chop and add to soups and stews. For a tasty side dish, stew trimmed beans in chopped or pureed tomato, sauteed onions and garlic. Season well and simmer until cooked through.

Green cabbage

Finely grate and saute with grated green apple and onion, then serve with pork sausages, or finely chop and add to soup. Make cabbage rolls by boiling cabbage leaves until soft, then rinse and set aside to dry and cool. Spoon a little Moroccan spice quinoa (see page 121) into the centre of the leaves and roll up to enclose. Add to a pan of pureed tomato and onion, seam-side down, then pour in enough water to cover and simmer until warmed through.

Kale, spinach, silverbeet, chard

Coarsely chop and add to soups. Steam and finely dice, then add to a tomato sauce (see page 227), or steam the leaves and saute in butter and bacon bits. Use the leaves like cabbage leaves to make stuffed rolls (see above).

Zucchini (courgettes)

Roast with other vegetables, finely chop and add to soups, or grate and add to meatballs (see page 164) or patties. Grate and add to whisked eggs to make an omelette.

STEAMED GREENS

Steaming is a simple, healthy way to cook your greens and brings out the natural flavour in just about any vegetable, from broccoli, asparagus and brussels sprouts to chard, kale and Asian greens. Trim your choice of vegetables and cut into even-sized pieces. Fill a large saucepan with 2–3 cm water, add the vegetables and cover with a lid. You don't want all the vegetables submerged in the water – there should just be enough to stop the vegetables sticking to the base of the pan. Bring the water to a simmer, which will create steam in the pan, and cook until the vegetables are brightly coloured and just tender, but still have a bite. The cooking time will vary but it should take around 7 minutes. (Alternatively use a steamer.) Toss the hot vegetables in a dressing (see page 116) or a simple mixture of olive oil, lemon juice, natural salt and freshly cracked pepper.

Beetroot is traditionally considered a blood and liver tonic and is wonderful for circulation, bringing a healthy blush to the cheeks.

Reserve the beet leaves to make another warm salad dish (see page 106).

Fresh beetroot, egg and rocket salad

SERVES *4–6 as a side*   **PREP TIME** *10 minutes*   **COOKING TIME** *15 minutes*

6 eggs
4 beetroot with leaves
2 handfuls of rocket leaves
    (or any lettuce leaf)
natural salt and freshly cracked pepper
Orange mustard yoghurt dressing
    (see page 117)

1. Immerse the eggs in boiling water for 5 minutes, then remove and cool under cold running water to stop the cooking process.

2. Cut off the beet leaves and set aside. Quarter the beetroots and place in a saucepan of boiling salted water. Cook for 10 minutes or until tender (test by piercing them with a fork). Remove the beetroot quarters and leave to cool. Strain the liquid into a jug and set aside.

3. Arrange the beetroot on a bed of rocket leaves. Peel and halve the eggs and add to the salad. Season to taste, then toss through the dressing just before serving.

TIPS: Drink the refreshing beet liquid with ice or as a hot drink, adding a squeeze of lemon juice for a tangy citrus twist.

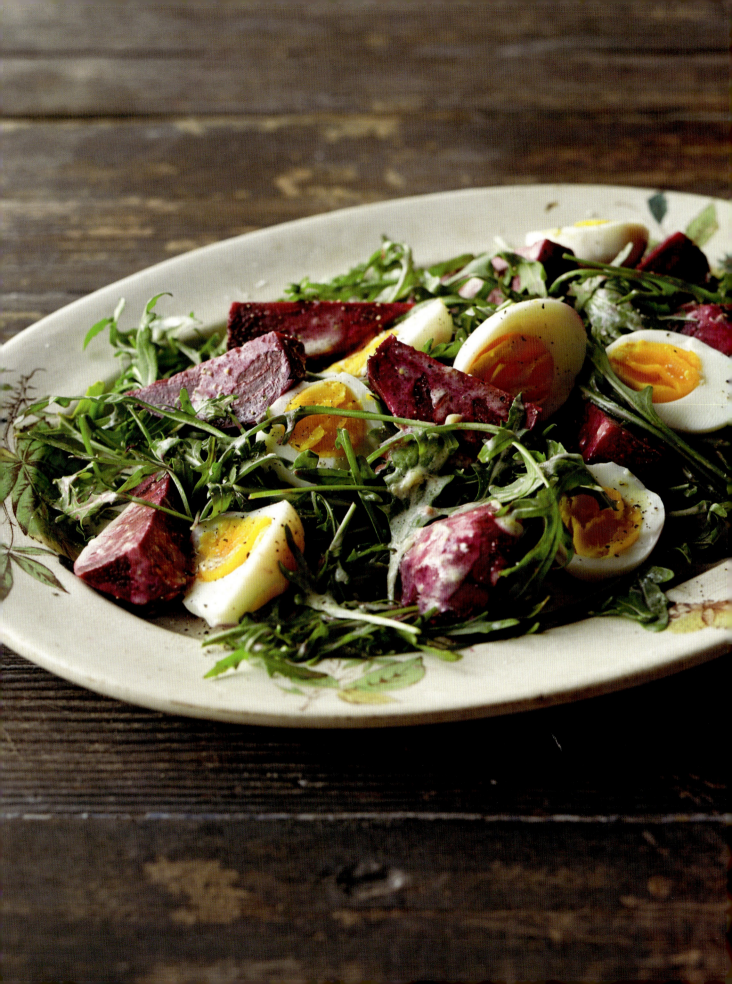

Beet leaves must always be cooked before consumption as they are high in oxalates, a type of plant acid that can bind to calcium and iron. Cooking reduces this effect.

Beet leaves with activated walnuts and olive oil and lemon dressing

Serves 4 as a side   **PREP TIME:** *5 minutes*   **COOKING TIME:** *7 minutes*

beet leaves cut from whole beetroots (see page 104)
Olive oil and lemon dressing (see page 117), to serve
handful of activated walnuts

1. Blanch the beet leaves in simmering salted water for 7 minutes. Drain, then dress with the dressing. Toss through the activated walnuts just before serving.

Fresh, lemony, crunchy and soft, this goes wonderfully well with fish or roasts. The bitterness of cos and radicchio stimulates healthy digestive function.

Pan-fried radicchio or baby cos with garlic lemon tahini dressing ›

Serves 4 as a side   **PREP TIME:** *5 minutes*   **COOKING TIME:** *6 minutes*

4 radicchio or baby cos lettuce, halved
extra virgin olive oil, for brushing
Garlic lemon tahini dressing (see page 117), to serve

1. Heat a frying pan over medium heat. Brush the lettuce halves with olive oil and place, cut-side down, in the pan. Cook for 3 minutes, then turn and cook on the other side for 3 minutes. Transfer to a dish and drizzle with the dressing. Serve warm.

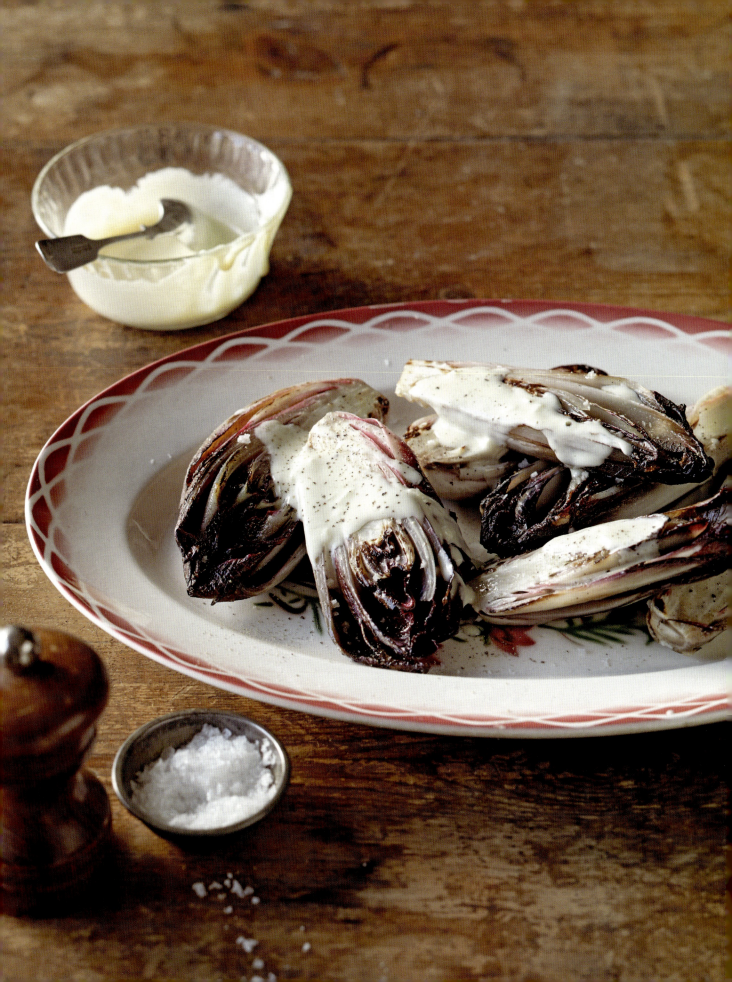

Zesty and sweet, this is a great side dish for lamb chops or roasts. The method of cooking carrots in butter allows for the conversion of beta carotene into vitamin A.

Orange butter carrots ›

Serves 4 as a side   **PREP TIME:** *5 minutes*   **COOKING TIME:** *10 minutes*

100 g butter
finely grated zest and juice of 1 orange (or use strips of orange rind, if preferred)
4 carrots, sliced
natural salt and freshly cracked pepper

1. Melt the butter in a frying pan, add the orange zest or rind, juice and carrot and saute over medium heat for 10 minutes or until cooked through. Season well and serve.

I am not sure whether the French eat this for health benefits or because it tastes so clean and healthy. Raw carrots cleanse the bowels, preventing the reabsorption of endotoxins. Endotoxins pollute the liver and blood leading to a hormonal imbalance or weight gain. Enjoy regularly as you would your greens.

Classic French grated carrots

Serves 4–6 as a side   **PREP TIME:** *15 minutes*

2 tablespoons lemon juice
½ teaspoon Dijon mustard
3 tablespoons olive oil
500 g carrots, peeled and grated
1 tablespoon chopped flat-leaf parsley
natural salt and freshly cracked pepper

1. In a small bowl, whisk together the lemon juice, mustard and olive oil until the dressing is completely emulsified. Stir the dressing into the grated carrots. Add the parsley and season with salt and pepper, then toss again and serve.

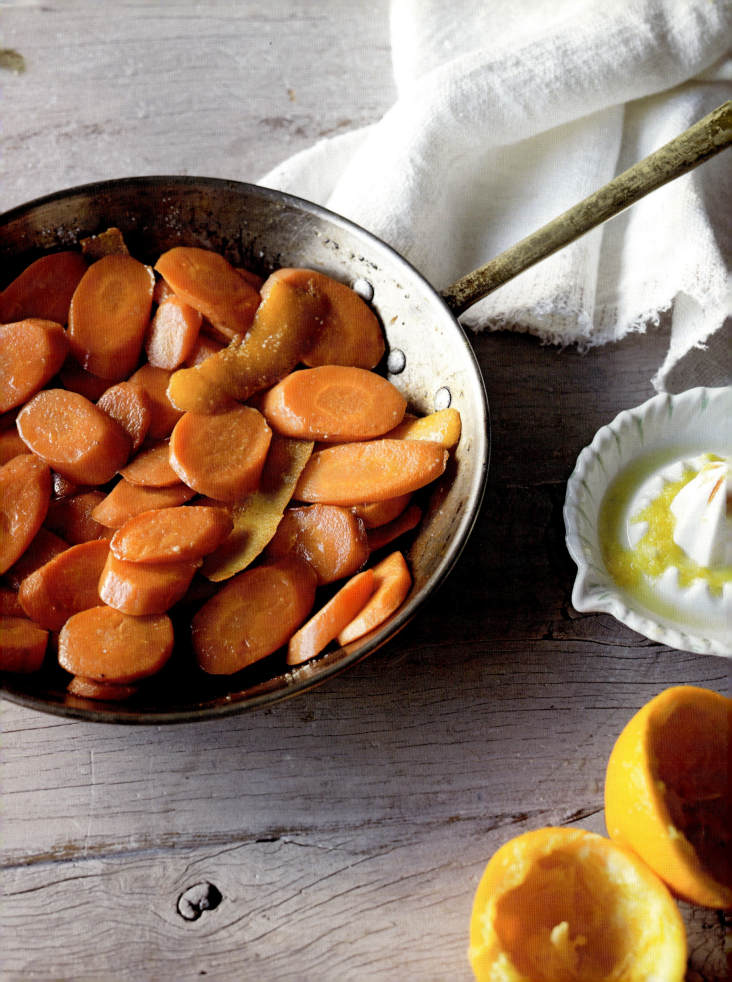

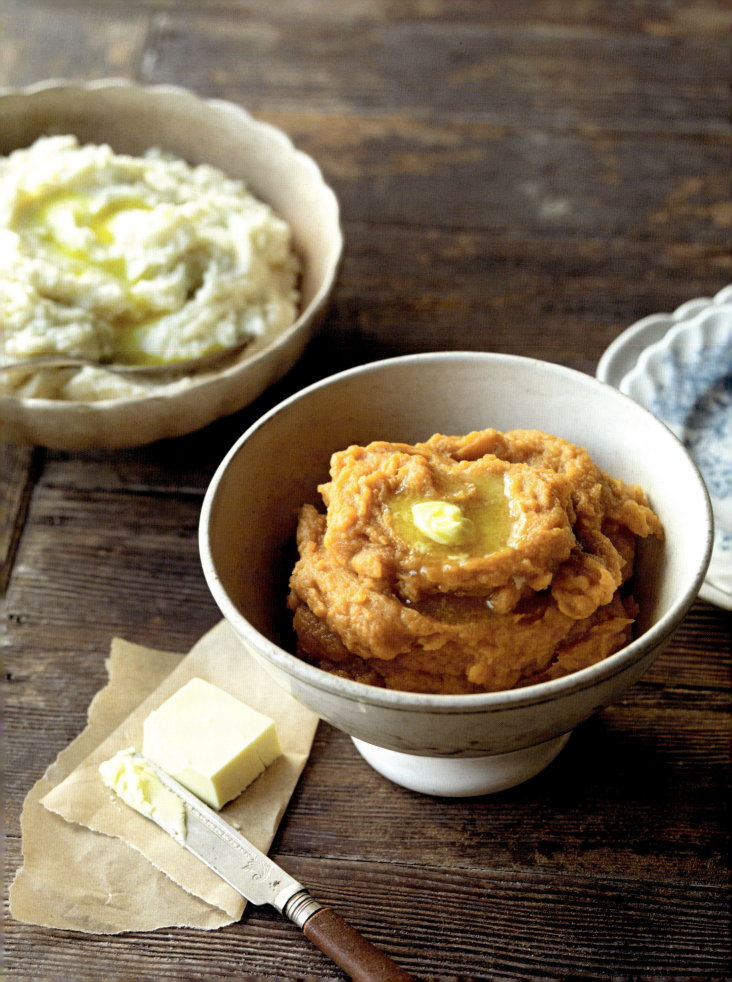

This mash is smooth, creamy and light, without the heavy starchiness of potato. For an extra creamy mash, add 3–4 tablespoons of fresh cream or ricotta.

Smooth cauliflower mash

Serves 4–6 as a side **PREP TIME:** *5 minutes* **COOKING TIME:** *15 minutes*

1 small head of cauliflower, roughly chopped
3 tablespoons extra virgin olive oil
60 g butter, chilled, roughly chopped
natural salt and freshly cracked pepper

1. Place the cauliflower in a saucepan of salted water and cook for 15 minutes or until soft. Drain, then transfer to a food processor. Add the olive oil, butter and salt and pepper to taste and process until smooth.

TIP: Cauliflower loves tahini. Serve steamed florets with Garlic, lemon and tahini dressing (see page 117).

This smooth and sweetly scented mash is the loveliest comfort food I know. Just like carrots, sweet potatoes are an excellent source of carotenoid antioxidants.

Sweet potato mash with cinnamon

Serves 4–6 as a side **PREP TIME:** *5 minutes* **COOKING TIME:** *15 minutes*

2 medium orange sweet potatoes, roughly chopped
1 tablespoon extra virgin coconut oil or butter, plus extra to serve (optional)
½ teaspoon cinnamon powder
natural salt and freshly cracked pepper

1. Place the sweet potato in a saucepan of salted water and cook for 15 minutes or until soft. Drain, then transfer to a food processor. Add the coconut oil or butter, cinnamon and salt and pepper to taste and process until smooth. Serve with a little extra butter, if liked.

LIGHT MEALS AND SIDES

This is one of those dishes that is different every time you make it, depending on which vegetables you have on hand. Choose from the selection below then proceed with the recipe. And always cook extra so you'll have plenty of leftovers!

Provincial roast vegetable salad

Serves as many as you like   **PREP TIME:** *10 minutes*   **COOKING TIME:** *35 minutes*

olive oil, for cooking
butter or duck fat (see page 159), for cooking
natural salt and freshly cracked pepper
2 tablespoons Provincial Herb & Spice Blend or dried rosemary, thyme and sage, to taste
lemon wedges, to serve (optional)

Choose from the following vegetables

onions, cut in half or quarters
garlic cloves or golden shallots, thickly sliced
tomatoes, cut in half or into quarters
parsnips, thickly sliced
swedes, cut into large chunks
turnips, thickly sliced
squash, cut in half
brussels sprouts, cut in half
green beans, topped and tailed
carrots, thickly sliced
beetroot, cut into quarters
celery, thickly sliced
pumpkin (squash), cut into chunks
fennel, thickly sliced
zucchini (courgettes), thickly sliced

1. Preheat the oven to 220°C (fan-forced).

2. If using onions, garlic, golden shallots or tomatoes, place them in a roasting tin, then drizzle with olive oil and add dollops of butter or duck fat. Season with salt and pepper and scatter over the spice blend. Place in the oven and reduce the temperature to 120°C.

3. Meanwhile, parboil the remaining vegetables in a large saucepan of boiling water until they start to soften. Remove them before they are fully cooked.

4. Remove the roasting tin from the oven and add the parboiled vegetables. Give them a stir, then return the tin to the oven and roast until the vegetables are golden, about 30 minutes.

5. Pile on a platter and serve with lemon wedges, if liked.

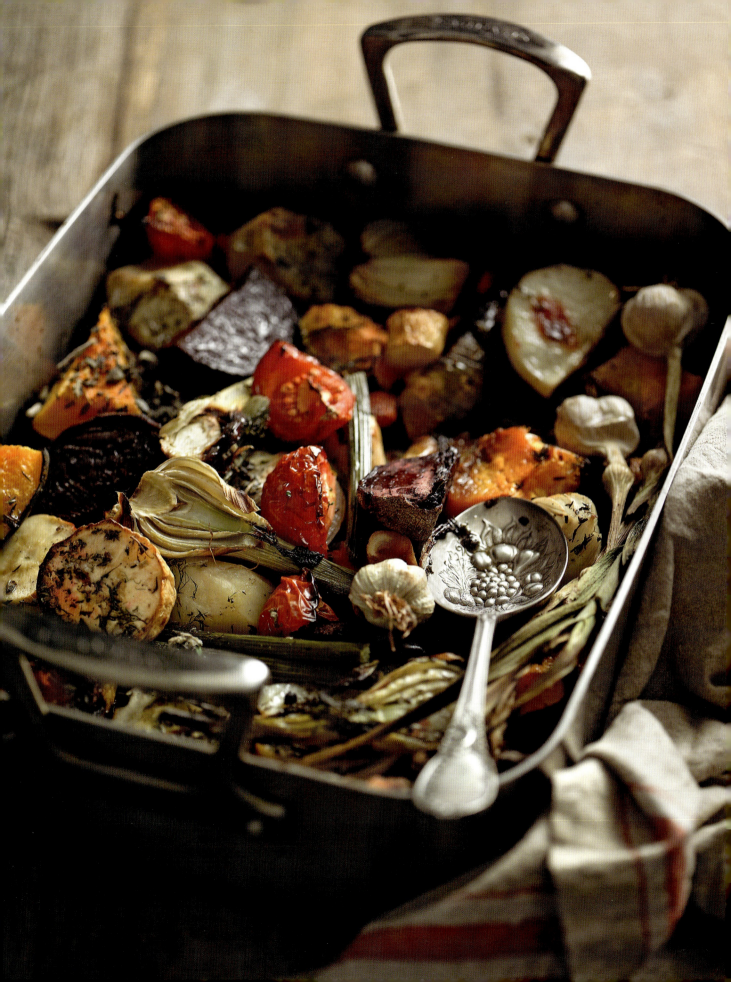

Quick Salads

All the salads serve 2 as a side dish

These fresh salads use simple ingredients that marry well when combined with a homogenous, flavour-enhancing dressing. Don't forget to chew, chew, chew your salads and vegetables – digestion begins in your mouth!

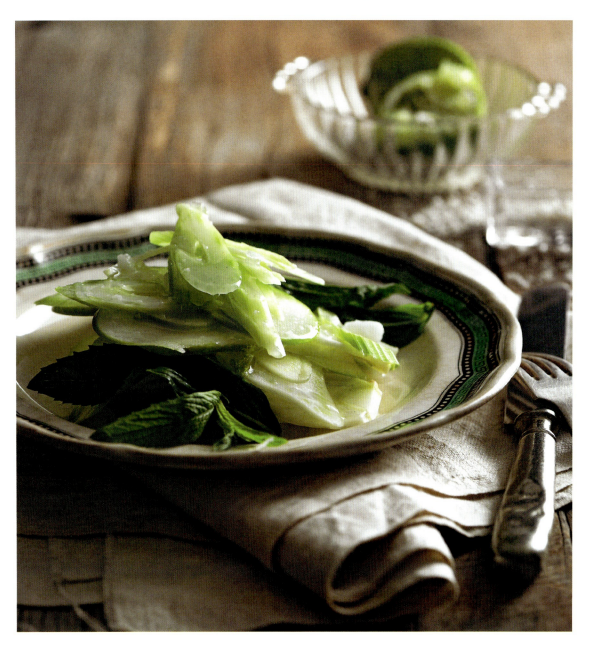

Apple, fennel and celery salad

This is one of my favourite salads. It tastes deliciously sweet and satisfying, but also freshens the palate and soothes the digestive system.

1 green apple, cut into quarters, thinly sliced
1 fennel bulb, halved, thinly sliced
2 celery stalks with leaves, sliced
10 mint leaves
Coconut oil and lime juice dressing (see page 117)

1. Combine the apple, fennel, celery and mint in a bowl. Add the dressing and gently toss to coat. Pile on a platter and serve.

Cucumber, ruby grapefuit and witlof salad

The gentle bitterness of the witlof and sweet tartness of the grapefruit stimulates digestive juices, which in turn enhance fat digestion.

1 thick Lebanese cucumber, thinly sliced
1 head witlof, leaves separated
1 ruby grapefruit, segmented
Olive oil and lemon juice dressing (see page 117)

1. Combine the cucumber, witlof and grapefuit segments in a bowl. Add the dressing and gently toss to coat. Pile on a platter and serve.

Leafy greens and herb salad

The fresh herbs in this salad offer vibrant antioxidants and chlorophyll to cleanse the body.

fresh herbs, such as basil, thyme, mint, flat-leaf parsley and oregano, roughly torn
lettuce leaves, such as cos, butternut, frisee and rocket, roughly torn
Olive oil and lemon juice dressing (see page 117)

1. Combine the herbs and leaves in a bowl. Add the dressing and gently toss to coat. Pile on a platter and serve.

Tomato with fresh curd and cucumber ribbons

Heirloom tomatoes offer a rich source of antioxidant lycopenes, a known anti-cancer nutrient. The longer the tomatoes are vine-ripened, the richer the antioxidant.

4–5 heirloom tomatoes, preferably a mixture of colours, sliced
1 thick Lebanese cucumber, cut into ribbons using a potato peeler or mandolin
200 g fresh curd (see page 216)
3 tablespoons extra virgin olive oil
3 tablespoons fresh lemon juice
natural salt and freshly cracked pepper
handful of thyme, basil or oregano leaves

1. Arrange the tomato and cucumber on a platter. Crumble over the fresh curd, then drizzle with olive oil and lemon juice. Season to taste with salt and pepper and finish with a sprinkling of fresh herbs.

Quick dressings

All the recipes make about ½ cup (125 ml) dressing

Dressings take no time to make but if you like to plan ahead they may be made on weekends and stored in containers in the fridge for up to four days. If you prefer a creamier dressing, consider using one of the dips on page 98.

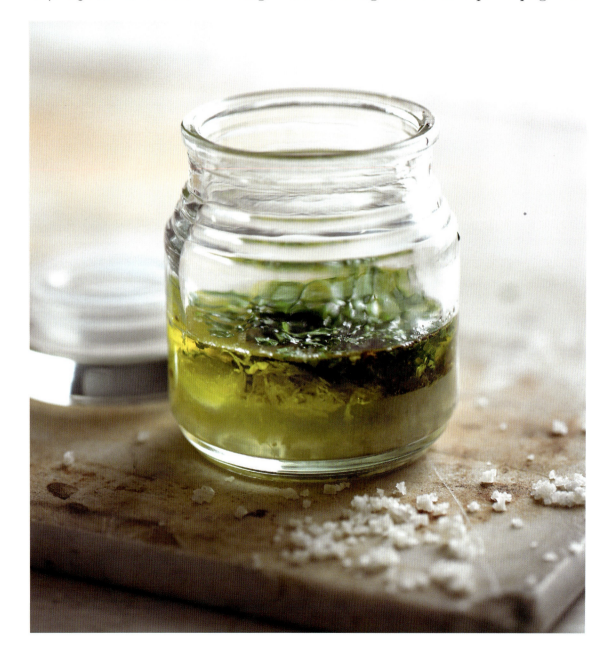

LIGHT MEALS AND SIDES

Olive oil and lemon juice dressing

3 tablespoons olive oil
½ teaspoon finely grated lemon zest
juice of 1 lemon
1 tablespoon finely chopped flat-leaf parsley, basil or oregano
1 clove garlic, crushed
natural salt and freshly cracked pepper

1. Place all the ingredients in a jar and shake well until they are emulsified. Taste and add more oil, juice or seasoning to your liking.

Coconut oil and lime juice dressing

3 tablespoons coconut oil
½ teaspoon finely grated lime zest
juice of 1 lime
1 stick of lemongrass, white part only, thinly sliced
1 tablespoon finely chopped coriander leaves and root
1 small chilli, thinly sliced, or to taste
½ teaspoon grated ginger
1 clove garlic, crushed
natural salt and freshly cracked pepper

1. If the coconut oil has set solid, melt it gently in a small saucepan.

2. Place all the ingredients in a jar and shake well until they are emulsified. Taste and add more oil, juice or seasoning to your liking.

Orange, mustard and yoghurt dressing

1 teaspoon wholegrain mustard
3 tablespoons yoghurt (see page 218)
3 tablespoons extra virgin olive oil
finely grated zest and juice of 1 orange
natural salt and freshly cracked pepper

1. Whisk all the ingredients together in a bowl. Taste and add more oil, juice or seasoning to your liking.

Garlic, lemon and tahini dressing

3 tablespoons hulled tahini
1 clove garlic, crushed
finely grated zest and juice of 1 lemon
natural salt and freshly cracked pepper
3 tablespoons extra virgin olive oil
1 tablespoon finely chopped flat-leaf parsley

1. Whisk all the ingredients together in a bowl. Taste and add more oil, juice or seasoning to your liking.

Fresh, green and rich in chlorophyll, beta-carotene and vitamin C, tabouli is a wonderful detoxifier and all-round immune booster. This is an excellent dish to serve with Lentil, lemon and garlic soup and Blackened eggplant dip (see pages 132 and 98).

Tabouli sans grain

Serves 4   **PREP TIME:** *15 minutes*

1 bunch flat-leaf parsley, finely chopped
½ bunch mint, finely chopped
1 large tomato, finely diced
3 spring onions, finely sliced
⅓ cup (80 ml) extra virgin olive oil
finely grated zest and juice of 1 lemon, or to taste
natural salt and freshly cracked pepper

1. Place all the ingredients in a large bowl and mix together well. Add more lemon for a zesty tang.

TIP: If you enjoy bulgur wheat in traditional tabouli, try amaranth as a grain-free alternative. Coriander can replace the parsley, if preferred, and red onion may be used instead of spring onion.

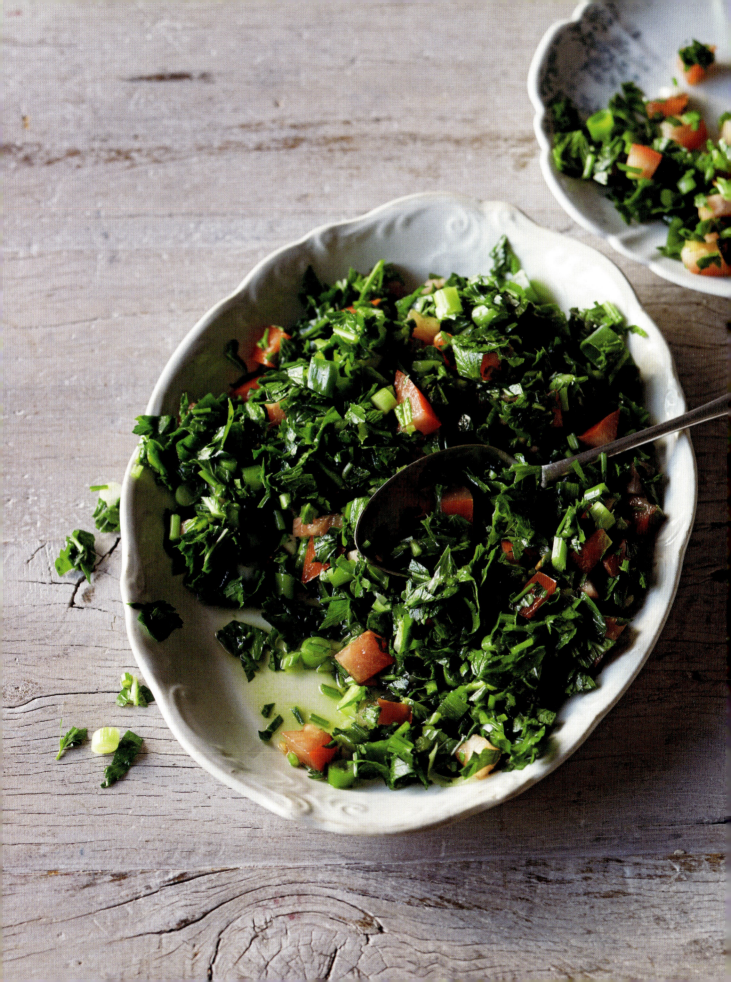

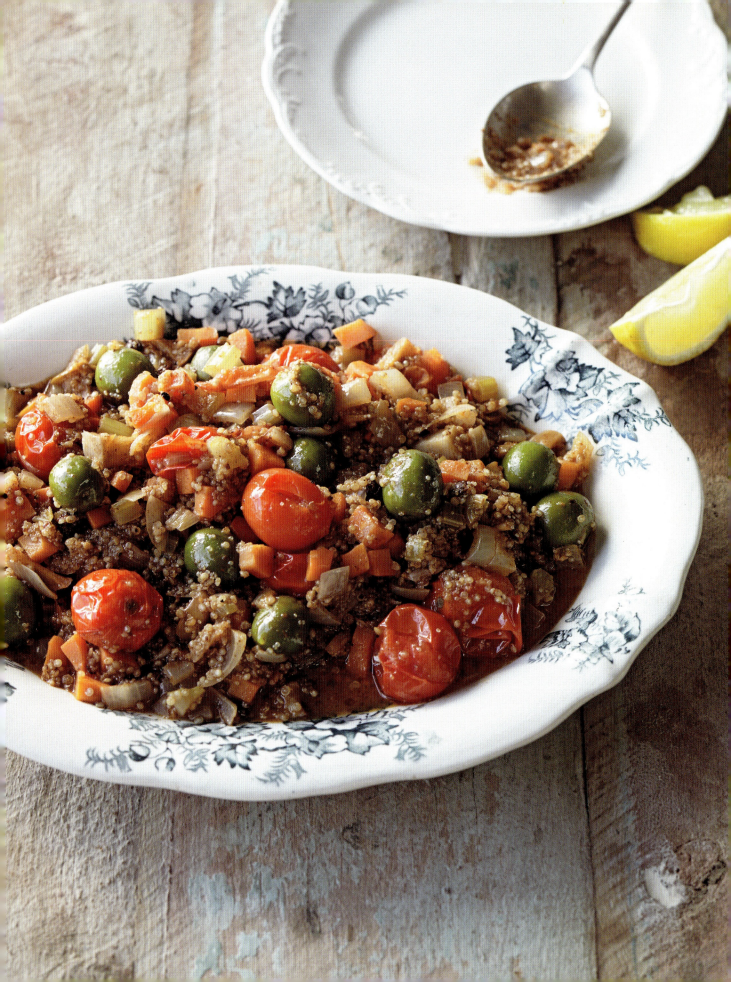

The tangy, tart and sweet flavours of this dish meld and marry beautifully with the nutty quinoa and amaranth, creating a vibrant tribute to the colours and aromas of Morocco. Start this recipe a day ahead to allow for overnight soaking.

Moroccan spice quinoa and amaranth

Serves 4–6 as a side dish **PREP TIME:** *10 minutes, plus overnight soaking* **COOKING TIME:** *15 minutes*

½ cup (50 g) quinoa and/or amaranth
juice of ½ lemon
natural salt and freshly cracked pepper
60 g butter
3 tablespoons extra virgin olive oil
1 brown onion, diced
1 carrot, diced
1 celery stalk, diced
1 cup (120 g) pitted large green olives
1 cup (160 g) cherry tomatoes
2 tablespoons ground sumac, sweet paprika, cinnamon and chilli powder, to taste

1. Soak the quinoa and/or amaranth overnight in 1 cup (250 ml) water with the lemon juice and a good pinch of salt. The next day, drain off any water and set aside.

2. Heat the butter and olive oil in a medium saucepan until melted and sizzling. Add the onion, carrot and celery and saute briefly over medium heat. Stir in the olives, cherry tomatoes, spice blend and salt and pepper to taste, then add the drained quinoa and/or amaranth and enough water to cover – about 1 cup (250 ml). Bring to the boil, then reduce the heat to low and cook, covered, for 10 minutes. Remove from the heat and keep the lid on for another few minutes to absorb the last of the liquid. Serve warm.

The level of omega-3 oils found in canned tuna is highly variable, as canning methods destroy much of the omega-3 oils in the fish. This is my alternative. It is an old Italian recipe I recall from my Italian neighbours when I was a child – the fragrant oil gently infuses with flavour as well as preserving the tuna. Some species of tuna are overfished, and wild tuna is always preferable to farmed. Due to their high position in the food chain, there is an abundant accumulation of heavy metals in tuna. By all means enjoy it, but eat it sparingly.

Tuna fillet in a jar

SERVES 2   PREP TIME *5 minutes*   COOKING TIME *5 minutes*

olive oil, for cooking and to cover
2 × 200 g tuna steaks, bloodline trimmed
1 bay leaf
5 black peppercorns
1 lemon, cut into wedges

1. Warm a frying pan over low–medium heat and add about 3 tablespoons olive oil. When warm, place the tuna steaks in the pan and cook just for a minute or so until they change colour. Turn them over and cook the other side – the middle will still be raw. Remove the pan from the heat and cover with a lid for 5 minutes. The tuna will continue to cook in the residual heat.

2. Put the bay leaf, peppercorns and lemon wedges in a medium sterilised jar, add the tuna and fill with enough olive oil to cover the tuna. Tightly close the lid and store in the fridge for up to 4 days. Just flake off what you want as you need it. The tuna is delicious in a salad or as part of a finger food plate (see page 86).

STERILISING JARS
Preheat the oven to 120°C (fan-forced). Wash the jars and lids in hot soapy water, then rinse and place on a sturdy baking tray (except plastic lids or rubber seals). Dry in the oven for 20 minutes. You could also use a dishwasher on the hottest cycle to sterilise jars, plastic lids and rubber seals. Dry well with a clean tea towel before use.

TIPS: Add your favourite herbs and spices to the jar to infuse the oil and tuna. Try chilli, lemon and garlic cloves or a teaspoon of Tuscan Herb & Spice Blend or dried oregano, basil and marjoram, to taste.

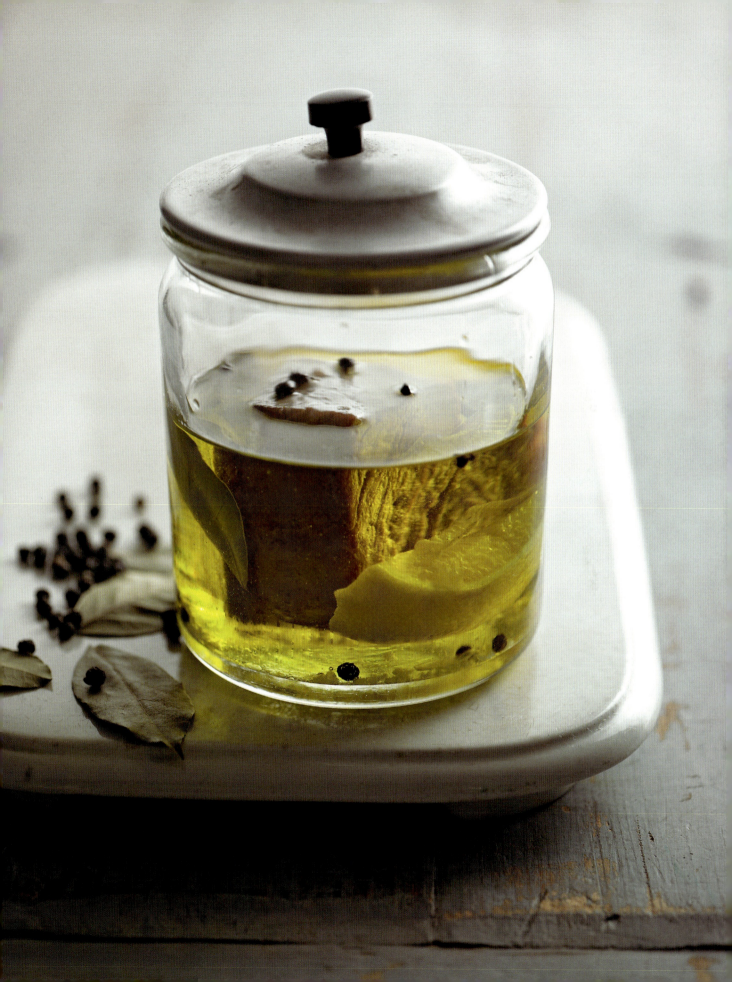

This can be made with a fresh or thawed frozen bone stock and the addition of a few simple ingredients. A clear broth is an excellent remedy for colds and flu, especially with lemon, garlic and some freshly grated ginger root. The addition of fresh or dried thyme and sage soothes a sore throat. A cup of broth as an appetiser before meals warms the digestive system.

Clear broth

SERVES *2 as a starter or side*   **PREP TIME** *10 minutes*   **COOKING TIME** *10 minutes*

2 cups (500 ml) fresh or thawed frozen bone stock (see page 214)
1 clove garlic, crushed
2 spring onions or 1 small bunch chives, thinly sliced
handful of flat-leaf parsley or coriander leaves, finely chopped
fennel leaf tops from 1 fennel bulb, thinly sliced
juice of 1 lemon
natural salt and freshly cracked pepper

1. Heat up the stock and garlic in a saucepan, then pour into a bowl and serve with the spring onion or chives, chopped herbs and fennel tops. Finish with a good squeeze of lemon juice for sharpness and freshness and season to taste with salt and pepper.

2. To turn a clear broth into a main meal, add your choice of chopped meat and vegetables. If you are not adding any meat, drop whole eggs into the broth – they will poach beautifully in the hot soup. Serve while the egg yolks are still soft.

TIP: The addition of dried seaweed to a clear broth adds more nutrition, such as iodine, and intensifies the flavours. Simply cut kombu or kelp, dulse, wakame or nori into pieces with kitchen scissors and stir into the broth until softened.

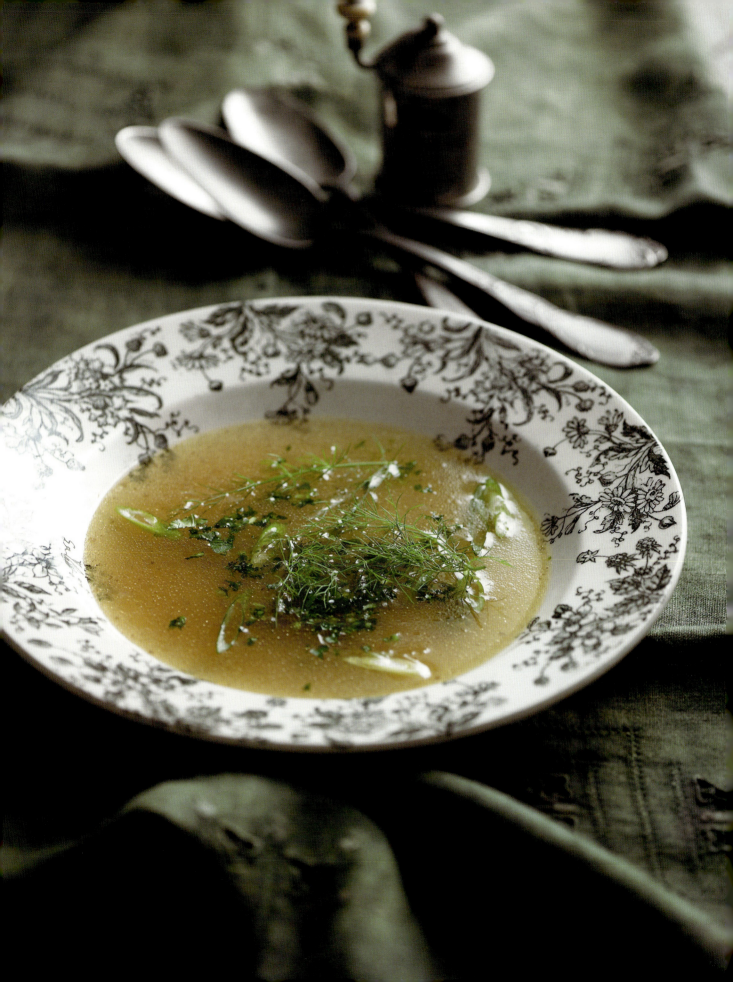

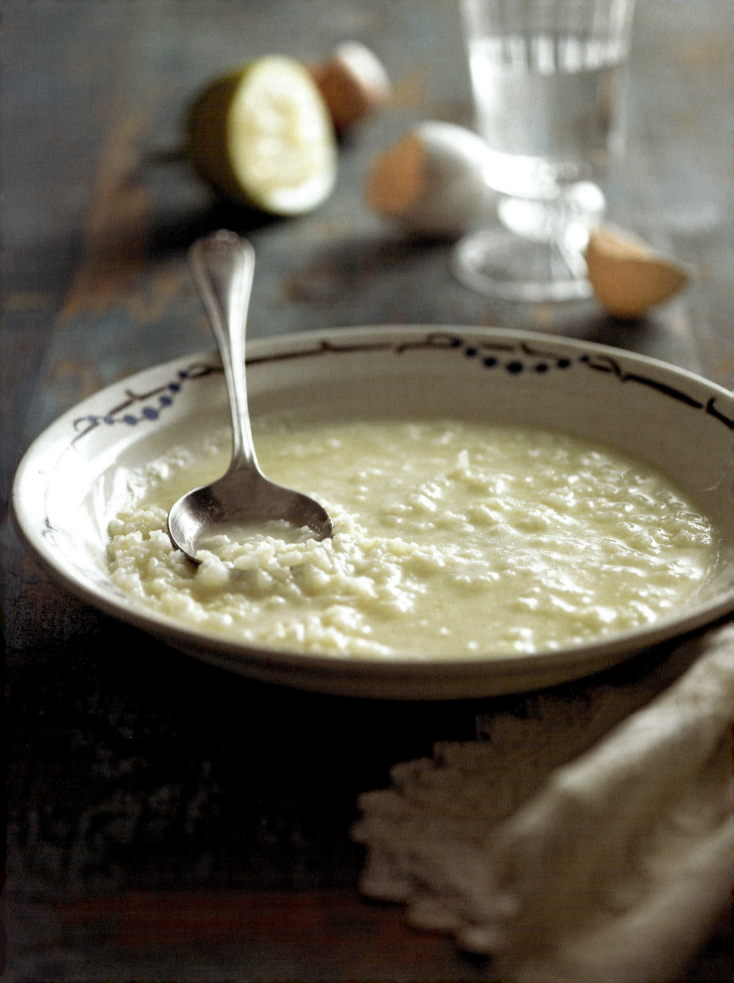

This traditional Cypriot soup is one of my favourite things to eat. It represents nourishment and is generally made for festive days, birthdays, family arrivals or when someone is feeling unwell – a medicinal soup for the heart and soul. It is made by boiling a whole chicken (use a boiler hen for real chicken flavour and nutritional density) or with homemade chicken stock (see page 214). The rice is not compulsory and the soup is just as delicious without it.

Chicken, egg and lemon soup

Serves 6 **PREP TIME:** *10 minutes* **COOKING TIME:** *2 hours 10 minutes*

1.5 kg chicken
½ lemon
natural salt and freshly cracked pepper
¾ cup (150 g) medium-grain white rice
3 eggs
½ cup (125 ml) fresh lemon juice, plus extra to serve

1. Wash the chicken inside and out, then rub with the lemon half and place in a large saucepan. Add 3.5 litres water and ¼ teaspoon salt. Bring to the boil over medium heat, then reduce the heat to low and simmer for about 2 hours or until cooked. Skim the surface of the water to remove any froth.

2. When the chicken is ready, remove it from the pan and place on a plate. Cover with baking paper and foil to keep it warm. Leave the broth simmering on the stove top. Add the rice to the broth and cook for 7 minutes.

3. In the meantime, place the eggs and lemon juice in a large heatproof bowl and beat until white and fluffy.

4. This next part of the recipe is very important to prevent the egg from curdling. Add 1 ladleful of rice soup at a time to the egg and lemon mixture, beating constantly. Continue adding the soup until the bowl is full. Then pour the egg and lemon mixture into any remaining soup in the pan and stir well to combine. Remove from the heat and serve with extra lemon juice and salt and pepper, to taste.

VARIATIONS
If you like, flake some of the chicken meat and add it to the broth; otherwise refrigerate it for leftovers.

A boiled chicken can also be roasted. Simply coat it in butter and season with Sunday Roast Blend or dried rosemary, thyme, sage and oregano, to taste, then roast in a preheated 180°C (fan-forced) oven for 20 minutes or until the skin is nicely browned.

Stracciatella, the Italian equivalent of this soup, is prepared by beating eggs with grated parmesan cheese, salt, pepper and nutmeg and then adding this mixture to simmering bone stock. The broth is set whirling first with a whisk, and the beaten egg mixture is added in a slow stream to produce the stracciatelle ('little shreds') of cooked egg in the broth.

This heavenly Thai-inspired soup can be made from a base of fish or seafood stock. If you like, you can make it with chicken bone stock (see page 214) and add chicken thigh fillets instead of the seafood. The fresh coconut and aromatic herbs and spices offer antimicrobial, anti-inflammatory and healing benefits.

Fragrant coconut soup with seafood

Serves 4–6 **PREP TIME:** *20 minutes* **COOKING TIME:** *25 minutes*

2 tablespoons coconut oil
1 large onion, finely chopped
2 cloves garlic, crushed
2 celery stalks and leaves, washed and cut into bite-sized chunks
2 large carrots, cut into bite-sized chunks
1 tablespoon sliced ginger root
1 tablespoon sliced galangal root
2 sticks of lemongrass, sliced
½ head of broccoli, broken into florets
2 zucchini (courgettes), sliced
2 kaffir lime leaves, thinly sliced
juice of 2 small limes
500 g fresh cleaned prawns, scallops, mussels or marinara seafood mix
2 cups (500 ml) frozen fish or seafood stock (see page 214), thawed
2 cups (500 ml) pureed fresh young coconut flesh and water (puree in a food processor)
natural salt

Garnish

finely grated zest of 1 lime
2 teaspoons coriander leaves
freshly cracked pepper
2 small chillies, sliced

1. Heat the coconut oil in a large stockpot over medium heat, add the onion and garlic and cook gently until they begin to soften. Add the celery, carrot, ginger, galangal and lemongrass and cook for another 5 minutes. Stir in the broccoli, zucchini, lime leaves, juice and seafood, then add the stock and coconut puree and a little water if needed. Simmer for 15 minutes or until the vegetables are soft and seafood is just cooked. Season to taste with salt, then top with the garnish and serve immediately.

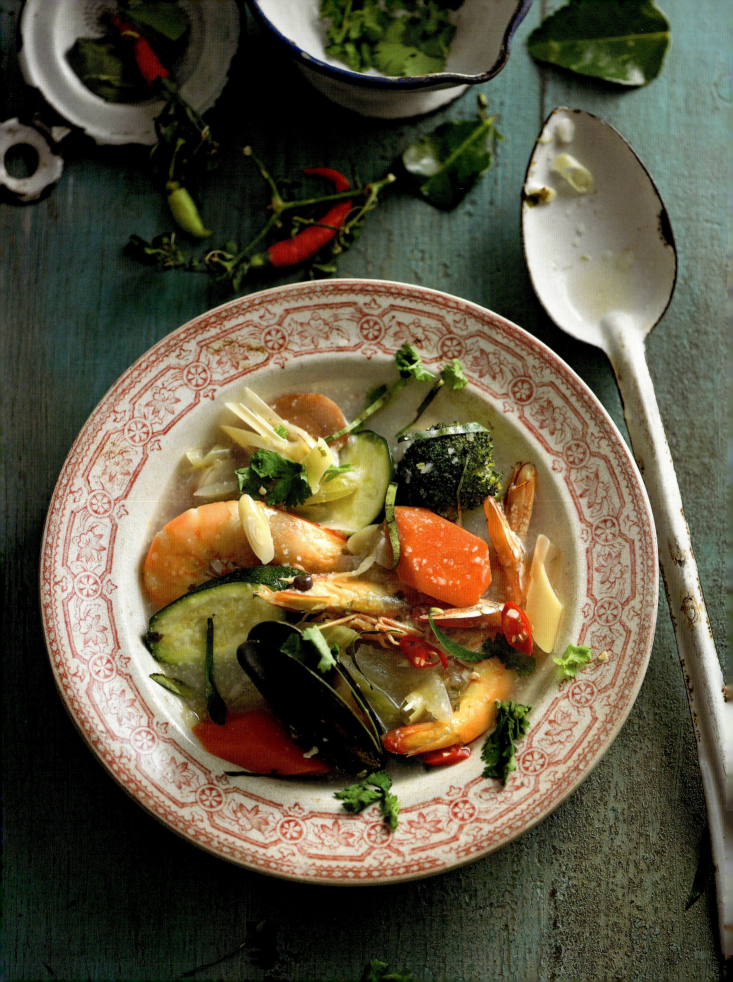

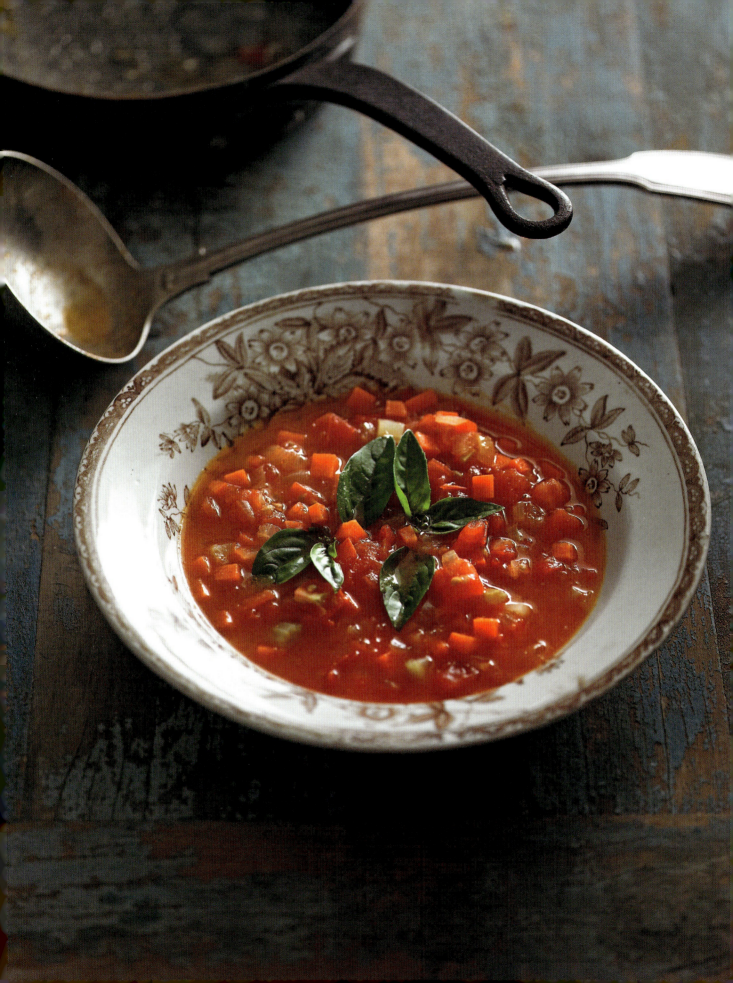

The base for any vegetable soup is a mirepoix (diced carrot, celery and onion) and a bone stock. A bone stock adds flavour and nutrition, and stimulates digestion and assimilation of the nutrients present in the vegetables.

Vegetable soup

Serves 4 as a side or starter   **PREP TIME:** *10 minutes*   **COOKING TIME:** *20 minutes*

2 tablespoons olive oil
40 g butter
1 onion, diced
2 cloves garlic, crushed
1 carrot, diced
1 celery stalk, diced
any additional vegetables you want to add
1.5–2 litres bone stock (see page 214)
natural salt and freshly cracked pepper

1. Heat the olive oil and butter in a large saucepan over medium heat.

2. When melted and sizzling, add the onion and garlic and cook, covered, for 5 minutes or until transparent. Add the carrot and celery and cook for a further 5 minutes or until the vegetables are tender. Saute any extra vegetables you want to add, then add the stock and season well with salt and pepper. Cover and bring to the boil, then reduce the heat and simmer until all the vegetables are cooked. Ladle into bowls and serve.

VARIATIONS
By simply adding extra vegetables and seasonings you can create any number of delicious vegetable soup combinations.

‹ Fresh tomato and basil soup
Add 2 cups (300 g) chopped tomato, a handful of basil leaves and 1 teaspoon Tuscan Herb & Spice Blend or dried oregano, basil and marjoram, to taste.

Pumpkin and ginger soup
Add 2 cups (500 g) chopped Japanese pumpkin and some freshly grated ginger and garlic. The pumpkin breaks up naturally or you can puree the soup for a smoother texture.

Leek and celery soup
Add 3 sliced leeks and an extra celery stalk, diced. Puree or eat as is.

Garnish
A fresh garnish can make all the difference to the flavour of a soup. Top soups with grated lemon zest, freshly grated parmesan cheese, a scattering of basil, flat-leaf parsley or coriander leaves or chopped chives, or natural salt and freshly cracked pepper.

A soup to strengthen and restore immunity, this peasant-style dish has equivalents in almost every culture. It is rich in antimicrobial properties, found in garlic and lemon. The lentils need to soak overnight so start this recipe a day ahead. Serve on its own or with a side dish of tabouli (see page 118).

Lentil, lemon and garlic soup

Serves 4–6 **PREP TIME:** *15 minutes* **COOKING TIMES:** *45 minutes*

100 g butter
1 onion, diced
1 celery stalk, diced
1 carrot, diced
3 cloves garlic, chopped
150 g green lentils, washed, soaked overnight (refer to page 212) and rinsed
1 litre chicken bone stock (see page 214)
1 tablespoon chopped flat-leaf parsley
juice of 2 lemons
natural salt and freshly cracked pepper

1. Melt the butter in a large saucepan or stockpot over medium heat. Add the vegetables and garlic and saute for 3 minutes or until the onion is soft and transparent. Add the lentils and cook for 1 minute.

2. Add the stock and 2 cups (500 ml) water and bring to the boil, then reduce the heat and simmer for 40 minutes. Stir in the parsley and lemon juice just before serving and season to taste with salt and pepper.

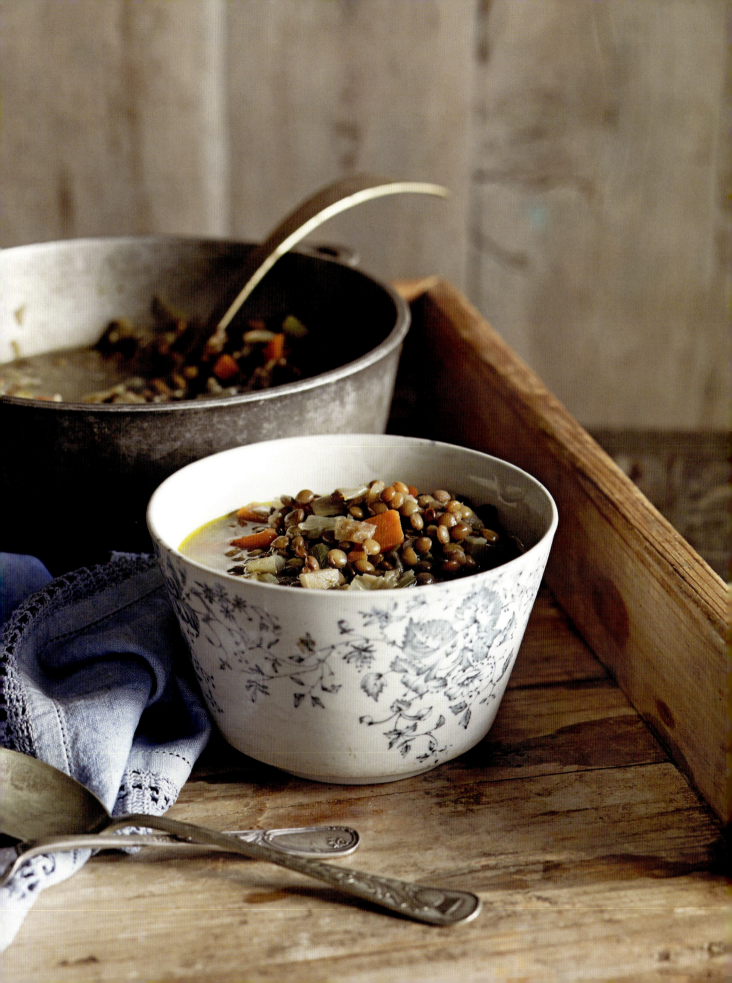

This eggy dish can be eaten at any time of day, cold or warmed up. It's a great way to use up leftover steamed or roasted vegetables, meatballs, chopped sausages and cheese, or you can cook the vegetables from scratch, as I do in this recipe. Lemon and egg isn't a usual combination but this comes from my Cypriot roots where we add lemon to absolutely everything we eat!

Lemon, capsicum and zucchini frittata

Serves 3–4   **PREP TIME:** *15 minutes*   **COOKING TIME:** *20 minutes*

40 g butter
⅓ cup (80 ml) olive oil
2 red or yellow capsicums (peppers), cut in half, seeded and diced
2 zucchini (courgettes), sliced
6 eggs
½ teaspoon finely grated lemon zest
natural salt and freshly cracked pepper
fresh lemon juice, to taste

1. Heat half the butter and olive oil in a heavy-based frying pan over low–medium heat. Add the capsicum and zucchini, then cover and saute for 10 minutes or until cooked. Add the remaining butter and olive oil, then whisk together the eggs and lemon zest and pour evenly into the pan. Season well, then cover and cook for a further 5–10 minutes or until the eggs are completely cooked. Serve with lemon juice.

This dish is made from raw minced beef. I had a brilliant one in the restaurant of the Musee d'Orsay in Paris and it is a memory I will never forget. I highly recommend you try this. Buy your meat fresh from a butcher who stocks grass-fed meats rather than pre-packed from the supermarket – particularly when using it raw. I like my mince freshly made on the spot so I know it's only meat and nothing but the meat. Raw beef – especially if grass fed – is rich in protein, B vitamins, vitamin D, iron, zinc and omega-3 essential fats.

Steak tartare

Serves 1 **PREP TIME:** *10 minutes*

200 g minced rib-eye beef, chilled
1 tablespoon capers, rinsed and drained
1 golden shallot, finely diced
1 teaspoon Dijon mustard
1 egg yolk
natural salt flakes

1. Combine the beef, capers, shallot and mustard in a bowl. Place a ring mould on a serving plate, and spoon the mixture into the mould. Remove the ring mould.

2. Make a small indent in the beef mixture with the back of a spoon and put in the raw egg yolk. Sprinkle with salt flakes and serve immediately. Make sure you mix the egg into the other ingredients so you get a bit of everything in your mouth.

Ceviche is essentially raw seafood marinated in lime juice. The proteins on the surface of the seafood coagulate slightly and appear to 'cook'. In a perfect ceviche, there is a balance of salt, citrus acid, onion, some heat and the fresh flavour and firm texture of the fish. The flavours are vibrant and stimulating and will have you salivating for more.

Prawn and scallop ceviche

Serves 2　**PREP TIME:** *15 minutes, plus marinating time*

8 raw prawns, peeled and deveined
8 fresh scallops off the shell
¼ small red onion, very finely chopped
½ long red chilli, thinly sliced
juice of 3 limes
1 tablespoon capers, rinsed and drained
½ small clove garlic, very finely chopped
3 tablespoons extra virgin olive oil
natural salt
witlof leaves, to serve

1. Wash the seafood in water and pat dry with paper towels. Using a very sharp knife, cut it into 2–3 mm pieces and place in a bowl. Add the onion, chilli, lime juice, capers, garlic and olive oil, then season with salt and mix well. Cover and refrigerate for 30 minutes for flavours to develop. Serve on witlof leaves.

TIP: Sashimi seafood is another way to serve raw fish. The best types are salmon, squid, shrimp, mackerel, tuna, kingfish, scallop and yellowtail cut into thin slices. Wasabi and pickled ginger are served with sashimi to add flavour and aid digestion, and also to kill off harmful bacteria and parasites that could be present in raw seafood. Rather than make it at home, enjoy sashimi at a great Japanese restaurant.

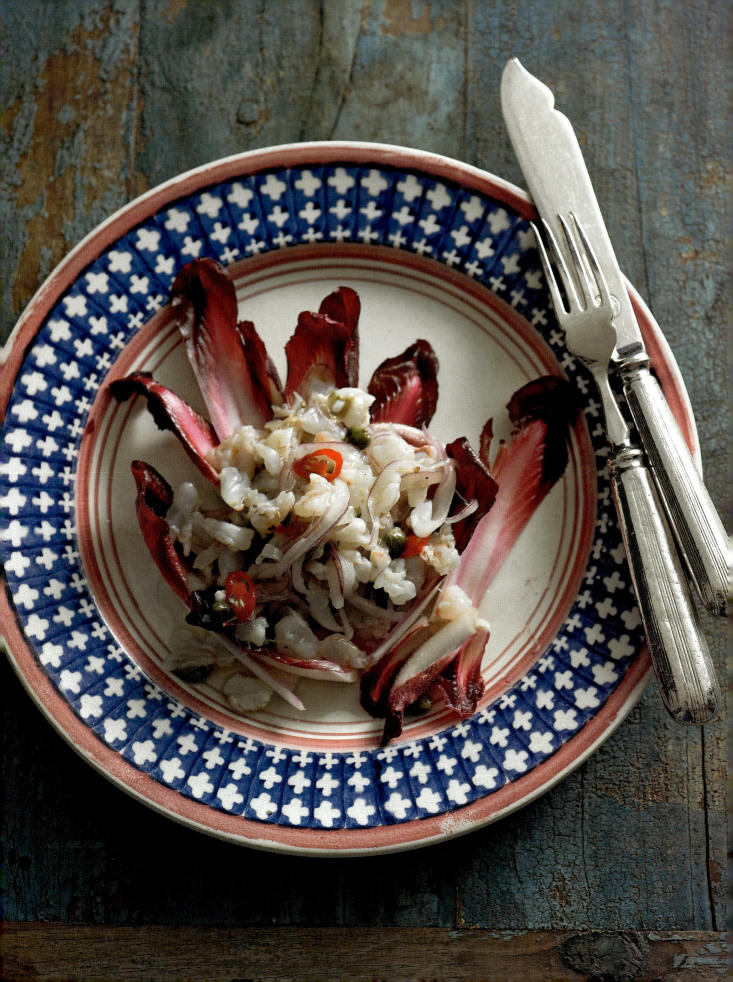

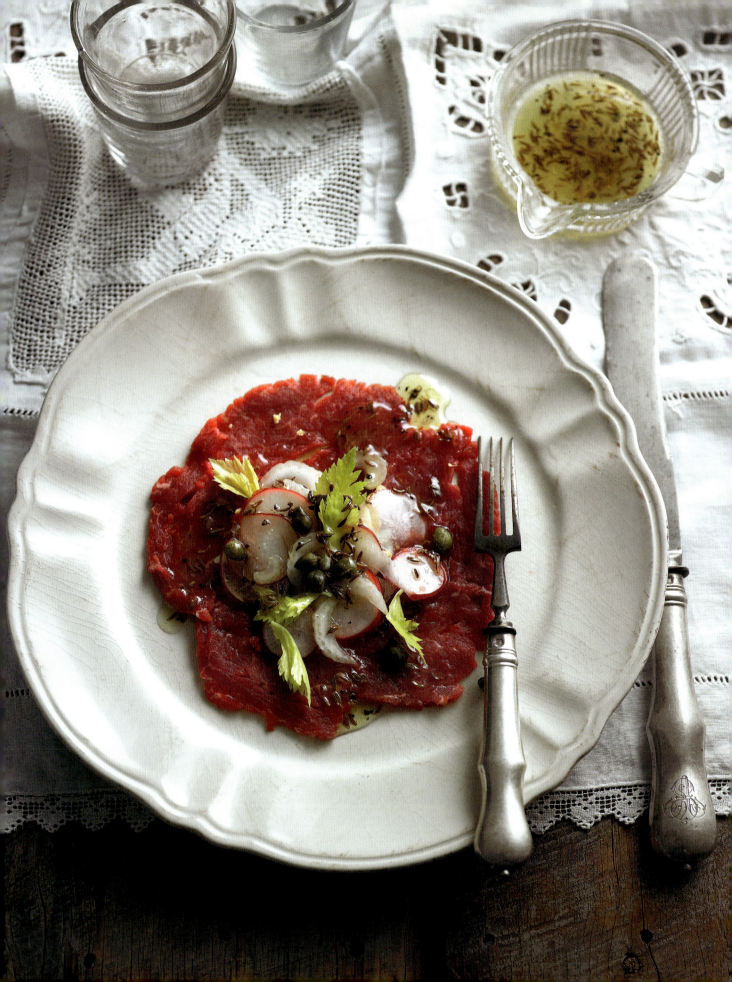

Carpaccio is a dish of raw meat or fish, such as beef, veal, venison, salmon or tuna, which is sliced paper-thin so it melts in your mouth. I'm using beef in this recipe, but you could replace it with raw fish such as wild salmon.

Beef carpaccio with radish and celery

Serves 2 **PREP TIME:** *15 minutes, plus chilling time*

---

200 g beef fillet, trimmed of sinew
4 radishes, trimmed
1 celery heart and pale leaves
90 ml extra virgin olive oil
2 tablespoons lemon juice
½ teaspoon caraway seeds
natural salt and freshly cracked pepper

1. Wrap the beef fillet firmly in plastic film to form a cylinder and refrigerate for 20 minutes or until firm.

2. Meanwhile, thinly slice the radishes and celery heart with a mandolin and roughly chop the celery leaves. Place in a bowl of iced water and stand until the vegetables are crisp.

3. Whisk together the olive oil, lemon juice and caraway seeds and season to taste.

4. Unwrap the beef and cut into very thin slices. Slightly flatten with the flat blade of the knife and arrange on serving plates. Drain the radish and celery, then place in a large bowl with half the dressing and toss gently to combine. Scatter the vegetables over the beef, then drizzle over the remaining dressing and season to taste. Serve immediately.

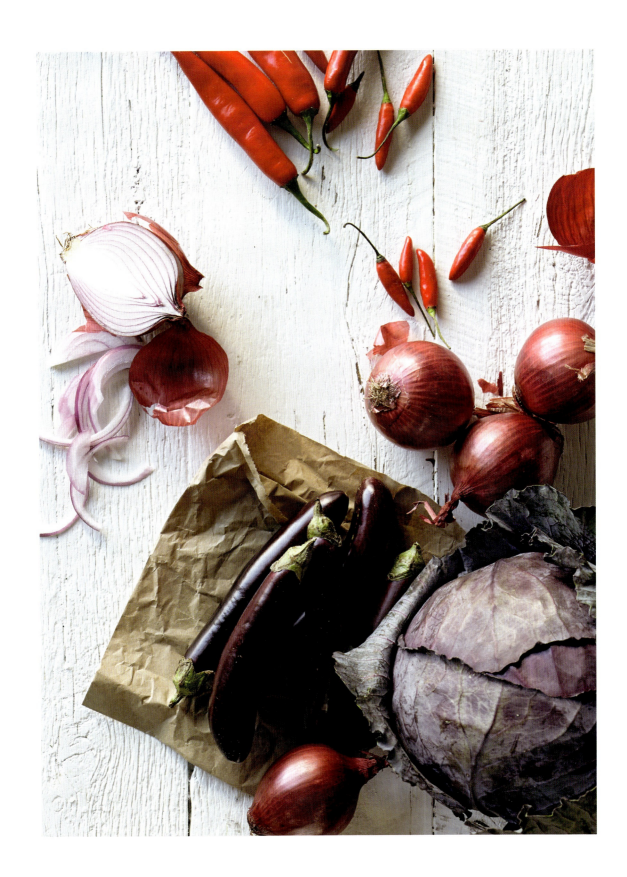

Dinner

After a long day at work, study or busy home life, cooking may feel like the last thing you want to undertake. Take-away might sound enticing but there is nothing like a home-cooked meal. The recipes in this chapter will hopefully inspire and encourage you to make delicious, nourishing food that brings happiness to you and your family.

If you get home at a decent hour, you can still create a meal in 30 minutes. The key is to have a well-stocked fridge and pantry full of fresh and dried foods. I also spend a bit of time on the weekend preparing a few basics (see pages 211–233) that will see me through the week.

What's for dinner when there's no time to cook? If there aren't any leftovers, choose one of the light meal options, such as a finger food plate (see page 86), mèze or antipasto platter – they all take less than 10 minutes to prepare. Pull together olives, dips, yoghurt, cheese, nuts, cultured vegetables, vegetables sticks, cherry tomatoes, cut fruit, boiled eggs or anything else you have on hand.

A slow food cooker is a genie in your kitchen as it cooks food while you are away. Put it on in the morning and a warm dinner will be waiting for you when you get home. Simply toss some salad leaves with dressing to serve with it.

But we're not always in a rush. This chapter also includes recipes for when you have more time to relax and savour each step of the preparation.

Lettuce makes an excellent wrap instead of bread if you are choosing to go without grains or gluten. Choose any lettuce leaf that is big enough to wrap ingredients in. I love iceberg lettuce because it is crunchy and fresh and has the perfect shape to cup your filling. Softer lettuces are better if you are rolling up your filling. Delicious fillings include leftover meatballs, roast lamb or chicken, raw fish, chopped egg, cheese or a combination of dips and cultured vegetables. You'll find recipes for most of these throughout this book.

Mexican fajita lettuce wraps

Serves 4   **PREP TIME:** *10 minutes*   **COOKING TIME:** *10 minutes*

1 teaspoon coconut oil
2 capsicums (peppers), cut in half, seeded and cut into thin strips
1 red onion, sliced
1 teaspoon Mexican Herb & Spice Blend or sweet paprika and cayenne pepper, to taste
500 g beef tenderloin, cut into strips
8 large crisp lettuce leaves
Guacamole (see page 99), to serve
½ cup (60 g) grated raw cheese, Cheddar, or other mild medium–hard cheese
1 bunch coriander, leaves finely chopped
thinly sliced red chilli, to serve (optional)
natural salt

1. Heat the coconut oil in a frying pan over medium heat, add the capsicum, onion and spice blend and saute until soft. Add the beef strips and give everything a good stir, then cook for a further 5–7 minutes.

2. Divide the beef mixture among the lettuce leaves and top with a big dollop of guacamole, some grated cheese, coriander and sliced chilli (if using). Season with salt and enjoy.

TIPS: Next time you have people over, set out bowls of fillings and toppings and plenty of lettuce leaves and let everyone help themselves. This is seriously moreish finger food.

If preferred, chicken strips or minced beef may be used instead of the beef strips.

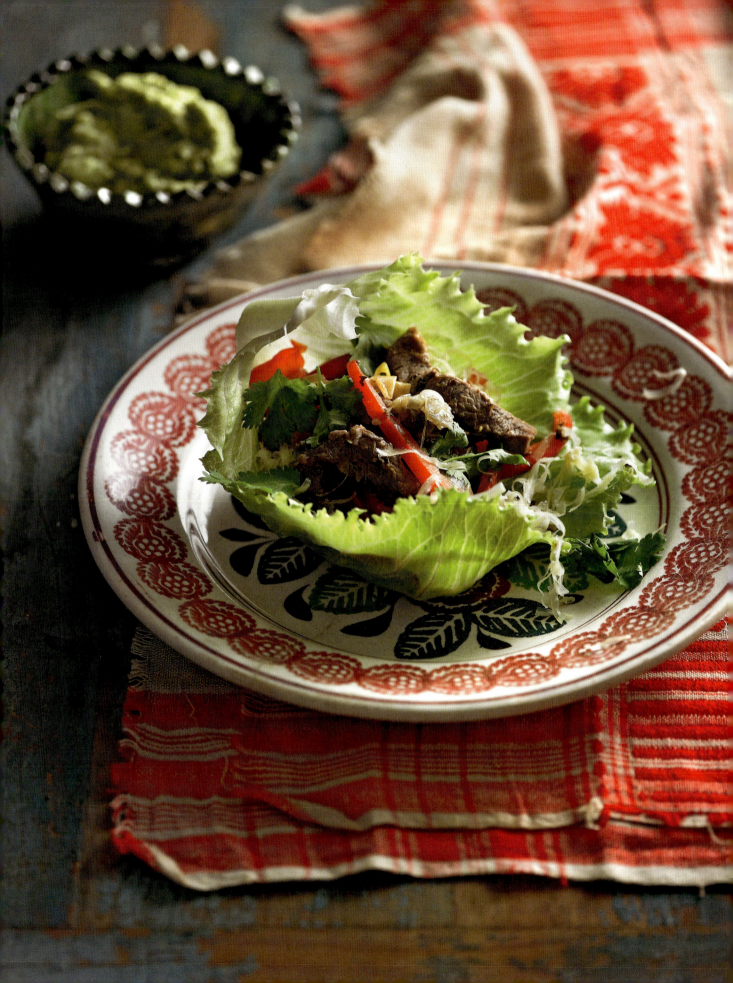

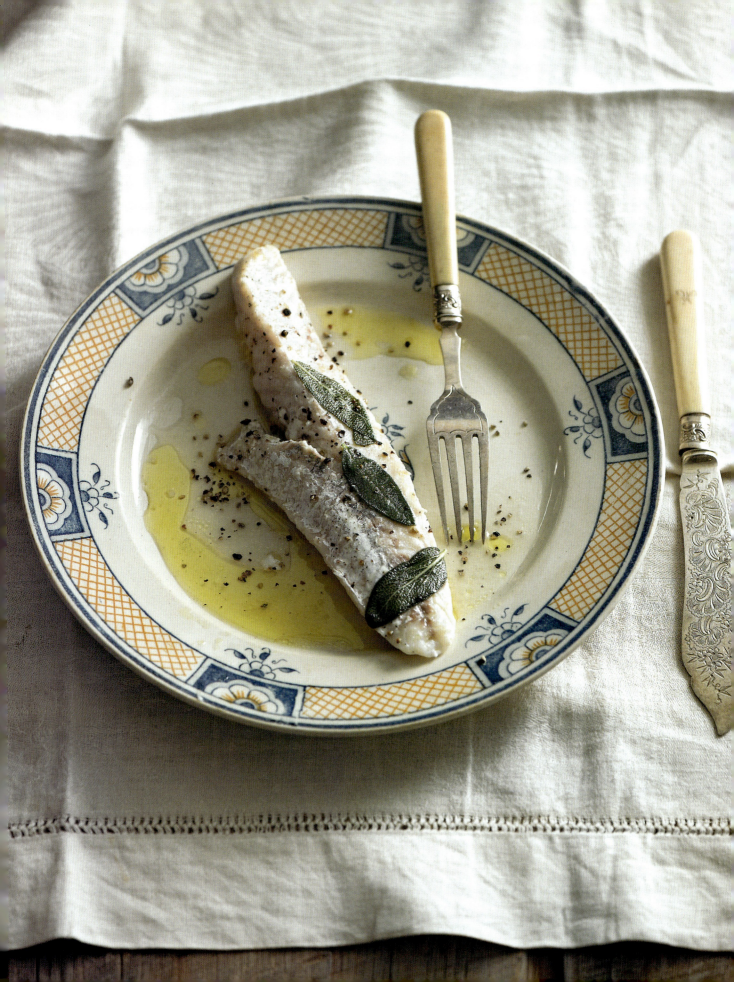

This is simply a fillet of white fish cooked in butter and sage and served with natural salt and pepper. It just melts in your mouth and doesn't need much else.

Fish fillets with sage and butter

Serves 4　**PREP TIME:** *5 minutes*　**COOKING TIME:** *10 minutes*

50 g butter, or to taste
8–12 sage leaves
4 × 200 g white fish fillets, skin and bones removed
natural salt and freshly cracked pepper
lemon juice, to serve

1. Melt the butter with the sage leaves in a large frying pan over medium heat. Add the fish fillets and cook for 3–5 minutes on each side until just cooked through. The exact cooking time will depend on the thickness of the fillet and the type of fish. Sprinkle with salt, pepper and a squeeze of lemon juice.

VARIATIONS:

Wild salmon fillet pan-fried in coconut oil and served with a crunchy Apple, fennel and celery salad and Minty cucumber yoghurt dip (see pages 115 and 98).

Whiting fillet pan-fried in butter and olive oil and served with green vegetables and Oven-blackened eggplant dip (see page 98).

Your choice of fish fillet cut in large chunks and pan-fried in ghee with scallops, prawns and Indian Herb & Spice Blend or a curry leaf and ground cumin, turmeric and fenugreek, to taste. Serve with steamed broccoli and cauliflower and Minty cucumber yoghurt dip (see page 98).

TIP: It can be tricky to know when a piece of fish is perfectly cooked. A tip I learnt from watching one of my favourite chefs is to insert the tip of a blunt knife into the fillet and leave it for 8 seconds. Place the tip of the knife on your lip. If the tip is cold, the fish needs more cooking. If it is warm, just cook a tad more, and if it is the temperature of a nice cup of tea then it is perfect! I like my tuna and salmon just under-cooked and pink in the middle. If you are cooking fish with skin, always cook the skin side first.

I grew up eating whole baked fish. My father used to go fishing and catch all sorts of things that he would simply bake in a roasting tin. Cooking a whole fish with the bone and head is so easy and has much more flavour than a fillet. The cavity is excellent for stuffing ingredients to infuse the fish with even more flavour from the inside out. Cooking for longer at a lower temperature is best, and you know the fish is cooked when it falls off the bone. Baking your fish in a dish it fits snugly into prevents it from drying out and the juices further infuse the fish with flavour and nutrition.

Baked fish with fennel, onion and parsley

Serves 4 **PREP TIME:** *15 minutes* **COOKING TIME:** *20 minutes*

1 lemon, cut in half
1 large fish (about 750 g), with head and bones, cleaned, scaled and gutted (or use 2–4 smaller fish)
40 g butter, diced
small handful of flat-leaf parsley leaves, chopped
natural salt and freshly cracked pepper
1 onion, thinly sliced
1 clove garlic, sliced
1 fennel bulb, cut in half and thinly sliced
2 tablespoons olive oil or coconut oil
Cucumber, ruby grapefruit and witlof salad (see page 115), to serve (optional)

1. Preheat the oven to 200°C (fan-forced).

2. Rub the lemon over the fish, then thinly slice the lemon. Stuff the cavity with the butter, parsley and lemon slices. Sprinkle with salt and pepper.

3. Arrange the onion, garlic and fennel evenly over the base of a roasting tin and place the fish on top. Season well with salt and pepper, and drizzle with the olive or coconut oil. Put the tin in the oven, then reduce the temperature to 120°C and bake for 20 minutes or until the flesh is falling off the bone. The cooking time will vary depending on the size of the fish. Cover with foil if you wish your fish to be steamed rather than roasted with a crispy skin. Remove from the oven as soon as the fish is ready and serve with cucumber, ruby grapefruit and witlof salad, if liked.

TIP: Choose a sustainable whole fish by consulting your local Marine Conservation Society. Ask your fishmonger to clean, scale and gut the fish for you.

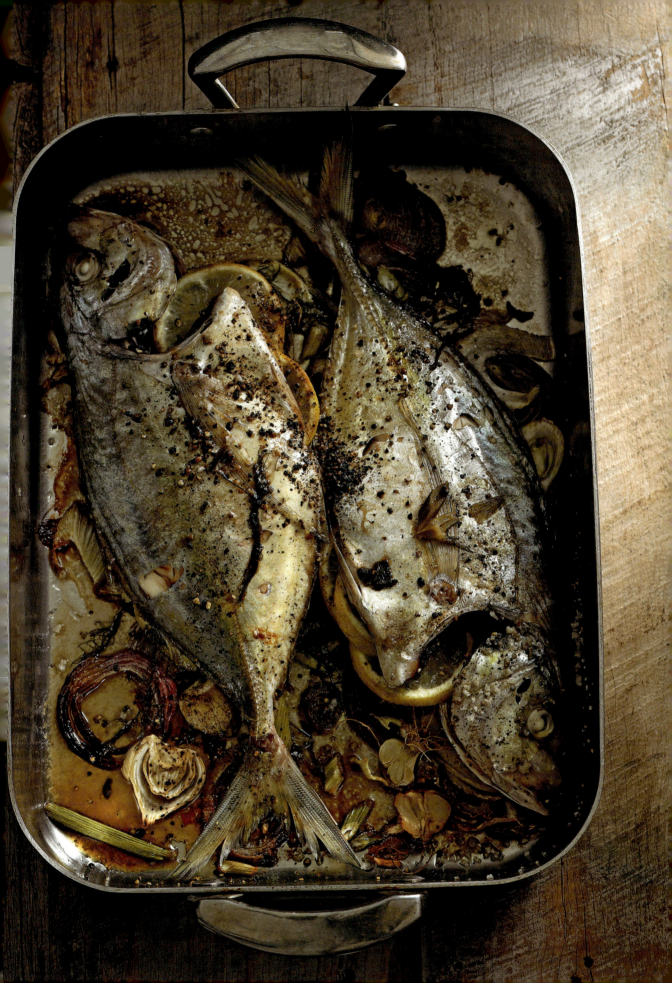

I love prawns and could eat them by the bucket load but I endeavour to source sustainable types as farmed, traul-caught or imported types are detrimental to our environment. I buy haul-caught School and Bay (Greentail) prawns – check out your local Marine Conservation Guide. This dish works well with peeled prawns, as here, but you could also use scallops, mussels or any diced seafood.

Pan-fried spicy prawns with cherry tomatoes

Serves 2 **PREP TIME:** *15 minutes* **COOKING TIME:** *15 minutes*

2 tablespoons olive oil
40 g butter
1 small onion, diced
1 clove garlic, sliced or crushed
1 celery stalk, diced
1 carrot, diced
½ teaspoon sweet paprika
½ teaspoon chilli flakes
natural salt and freshly cracked pepper
10 raw prawns, peeled and deveined
10 cherry tomatoes
Leafy greens and herb salad (see page 115), to serve (optional)

1. Heat the olive oil and butter in a frying pan over medium heat. Add the onion and garlic and cook, covered, for 5 minutes or until transparent. Add the celery and carrot and cook for another 5 minutes or until the vegetables are cooked. Season with paprika, chilli, salt and pepper. Toss in the prawns and cherry tomatoes and stir over the heat until the prawns are pink and just cooked through. Serve as is or with leafy greens and herb salad.

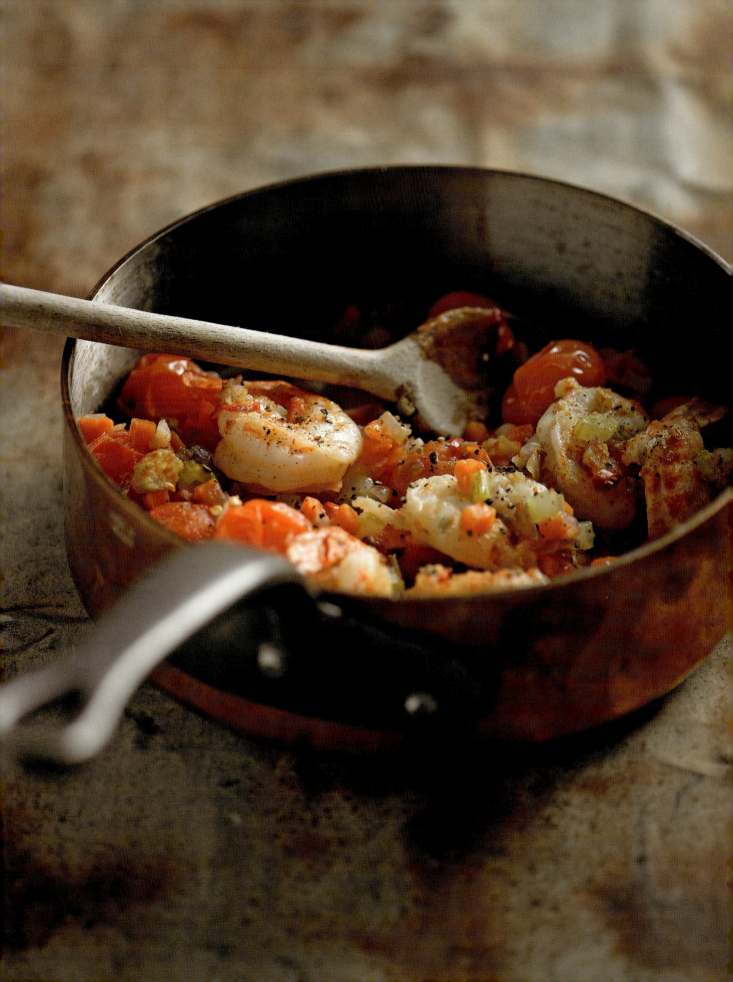

Sardines are rich in calcium and other minerals, and vitamins A, D and B12. They have lower levels of mercury and other pollutants than larger fish, such as shark and tuna, because they are so low on the aquatic food chain, feeding mostly on plankton. I prefer to eat fresh sardines rather than the canned variety as they are richer in nutrients and come without the detrimental plastics that line the cans.

Raw marinated sardines with zesty tomato

Serves 4   **PREP TIME:** *10 minutes, plus marinating time*

12 fresh sardines, cleaned and filleted (ask your fishmonger to do this for you)
100 ml extra virgin olive oil
1 clove garlic, thinly sliced
finely grated zest and juice of 1 lemon
1 ripe tomato, grated (discard skin)
½ teaspoon Tuscan Herb & Spice Blend or dried oregano, basil and marjoram, to taste
natural salt
sliced cucumber, to serve

1. Place the sardine fillets in a shallow dish.

2. Combine the olive oil, garlic, lemon zest, juice, grated tomato and spice blend in a bowl and season to taste with salt. Pour over the sardines, then cover with plastic film and marinate in the fridge for at least 30 minutes.

3. Transfer to a serving plate and serve with freshly sliced cucumber.

TIP: If preferred, the sardines can also be baked. Place them in a baking dish in a preheated 120°C fan-forced oven for about 15 minutes.

Baking is an effortless and healthy method of cooking a meal and fills the house with a warming aroma. By covering the baking dish with baking paper and foil, you create a little cocoon for the food to steam in its own juices. I don't cover the food directly in foil as aluminium can leach into the food. Remove the covering for the last 10 minutes of cooking so the food can brown nicely. Choose a baking dish made from stainless steel, ovenproof glass, cast iron or ceramic.

Baked fennel sausages with eggplants and tomato

Serves 4 **PREP TIME:** *15 minutes* **COOKING TIME:** *40 minutes*

1 onion, diced
2 cloves garlic, sliced
1 eggplant (aubergine), diced
4 tomatoes, diced
2 teaspoons fennel seeds
natural salt and freshly cracked pepper
8 sausages
cultured vegetables (see page 221) and Tabouli sans grains (see page 118), to serve

1. Preheat the oven to 200°C (fan-forced).

2. Place the onion, garlic, eggplant and tomato in a baking dish. Sprinkle over the fennel seeds and season well. Place the sausages on top of the vegetables.

3. Reduce the oven temperature to 120°C, then cover with baking paper and foil and bake for 40 minutes or until the sausages are cooked through (check by piercing with a skewer – the liquid that runs out should be clear).

4. Divide the sausages and vegetables among dinner plates, add a tablespoon of cultured vegetables (to aid digestion) and serve with tabouli sans grains.

TIP: I prefer to use grain-free sausages made from the best quality ingredients: minced meat, fats and fresh or dried herbs and spices.

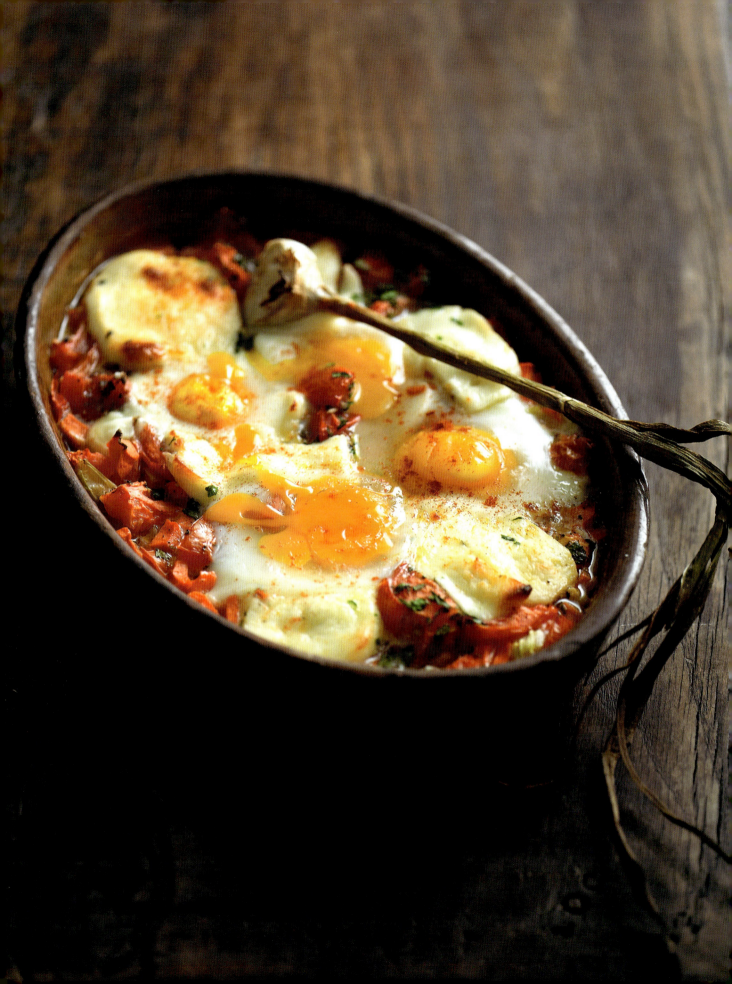

Haloumi is a Cypriot semi-hard, unripened cheese made from a mixture of goat and sheep milk, traditionally sprinkled with dried peppermint leaves and soaked in brine. The mint combined with the saltiness of the haloumi infuses the tomato base of this dish but what I love most is how the cheese softens without melting and squeaks between your teeth as you chew it. Haloumi is my choice for this dish but you could also use fresh curds (see page 216), bocconcini or mozzarella slices.

Baked eggs with tomato and haloumi

Serves 2   **PREP TIME:** *10 minutes*   **COOKING TIME:** *40 minutes*

40 g butter
1 celery stalk, diced
1 clove garlic, sliced or crushed
1 carrot, diced
2 cups (560 g) finely chopped tomatoes
handful of flat-leaf parsley leaves
natural salt and freshly cracked pepper
1 × 250 g packet haloumi cheese, cut into 1 cm thick slices
4 eggs

1. Preheat the oven to 220°C (fan-forced).

2. Grease a baking dish generously with the butter. Combine the celery, garlic, carrot, pureed tomatoes and parsley leaves in the baking dish and add a splash of water. Season well. Sit the haloumi slices on top.

3. Reduce the oven temperature to 180°C, then cover with baking paper and foil and bake for 20–30 minutes or until bubbling.

4. Remove the covering and make 4 indents in the mixture with the back of a spoon. Crack the eggs into the indents, then return the covering and bake for 10 minutes or until the eggs are cooked with a soft yolk. Serve immediately.

I only use pastured chooks as the care taken in their farming is reflected in the gorgeous, juicy quality of the meat. I ask for marylands (leg and thigh portions) and my butcher will bone the thigh. I keep the bones for a chicken stock and the legs for Spicy lemon butter chicken legs.

Chicken thigh fillets have more protein and general nutrients than a breast fillet. Thighs with bones are even more nutrient dense as the minerals in the bones impart their nutrition when cooked with the chicken meat.

Salt and pepper chilli chicken with lime ›

Serves 4 **PREP TIME:** *10 minutes* **COOKING TIME:** *20 minutes*

extra virgin coconut oil, for pan-frying
8 chicken thigh fillets
2 spring onions, sliced
2 small chillies, sliced, or 2 tablespoons ground sumac, sweet paprika and chilli powder, to taste
finely grated zest and juice of 2 limes
natural salt and freshly cracked pepper
Apple, fennel and celery salad (see page 115), to serve

1. Heat the coconut oil in a frying pan over medium heat. When the oil is hot, add the chicken thighs and cook for 10 minutes or until lightly golden. Turn them over and cook the other side for a further 10 minutes. Transfer to a large serving plate and scatter over the spring onion, chilli or spice blend, lime zest and juice and lots of salt and pepper. Serve immediately with the apple, fennel and celery salad.

Mmmmmmm . . . much like the lamb chops, these are best eaten with your fingers so you don't miss even a tiny morsel. Once you start, it's hard to stop!

Spicy lemon butter chicken legs

Serves 4 **PREP TIME:** *5 minutes* **COOKING TIME:** *40 minutes*

3 tablespoons extra virgin olive oil
60 g butter
8 chicken legs
2 teaspoons Mexican Herb & Spice Blend or sweet paprika and cayenne pepper, to taste
finely grated zest and juice of 2 lemons
natural salt and freshly cracked pepper

1. Heat the olive oil and butter in a frying pan over medium heat. When the oil is hot, add the chicken legs and cook for 15 minutes each side. Remove the pan from the heat, cover and let the chicken steam for a further 10 minutes. Transfer to a large serving plate and sprinkle over the spice blend, lemon zest and juice, and lots of salt and pepper. Serve immediately with plenty of napkins for sticky fingers!

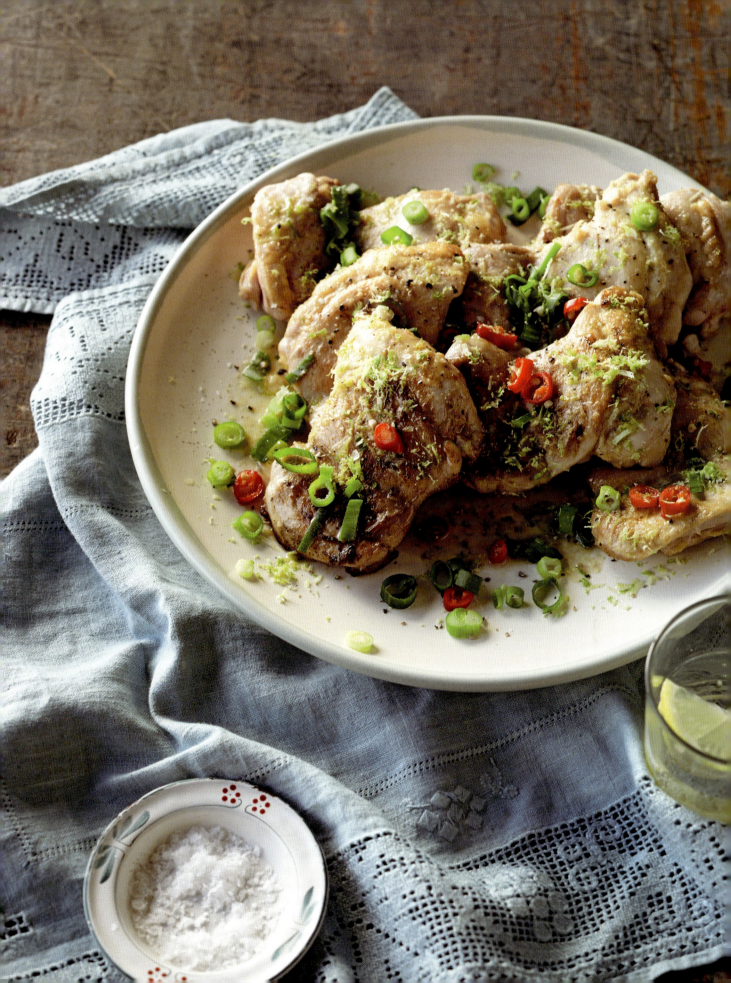

Like a slow-cooked curry, this dish is infused with Indian curry flavours but takes a fraction of the time to cook. For best results, use a heavy cast-iron or stainless-steel frying pan with a lid.

Indian spiced chicken with spinach

Serves 2 **PREP TIME:** *15 minutes* **COOKING TIME:** *40 minutes*

2 tablespoons olive oil
2 tablespoons ghee or butter
1 onion, diced
1 clove garlic, sliced or crushed
1 celery stick, diced
1 carrot, diced
6 chicken thighs fillets, cut into strips
1 cup (250 ml) chicken bone stock (see page 214)
1 teaspoon Indian Herb & Spice Blend or a curry leaf and ground cumin, turmeric and fenugreek, to taste
natural salt and freshly cracked pepper
1 cup (30 g) baby spinach leaves
Minty cucumber yoghurt dip (see page 98), to serve (optional)

1. Heat the olive oil and ghee or butter in a frying pan over medium heat. When hot, stir in the onion and garlic and cook, covered, for 5 minutes or until the onion is transparent. Add the celery and carrot and cook, covered, for a further 5 minutes or until the vegetables are cooked. Add the chicken strips and stir for a few minutes, then pour in the stock and season with the spice blend, salt and pepper.

2. Reduce the heat to low, then cover and cook for another 20 minutes. Add a little water if it starts to dry out. Toss in the spinach leaves and cook for another 5 minutes with the lid on. Serve with the minty cucumber yoghurt dip, if liked.

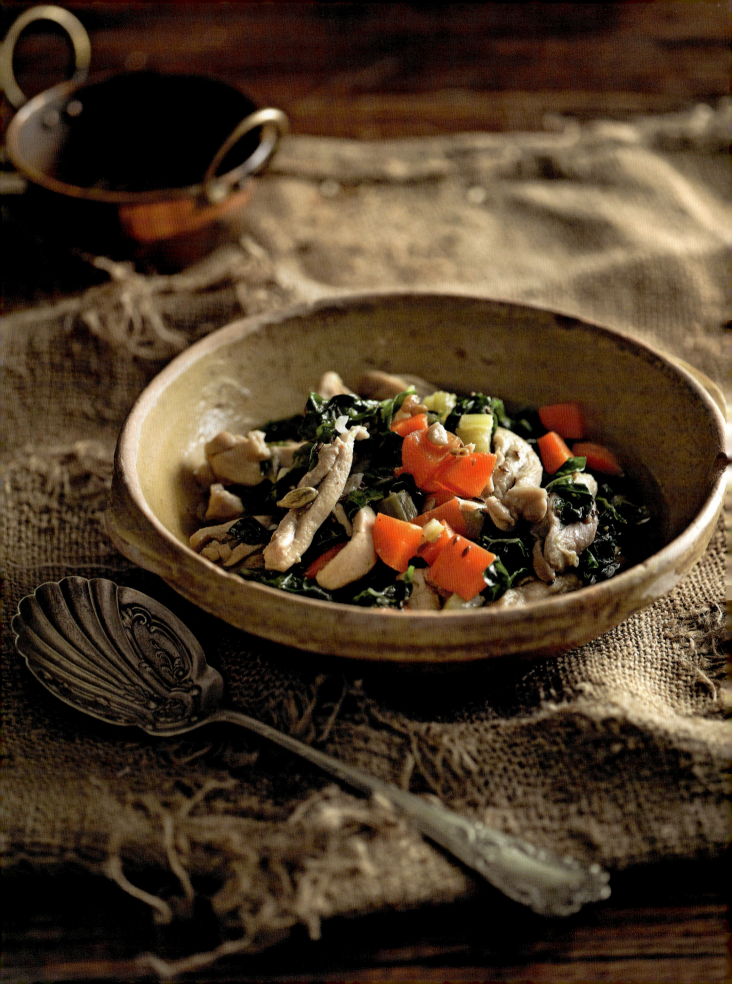

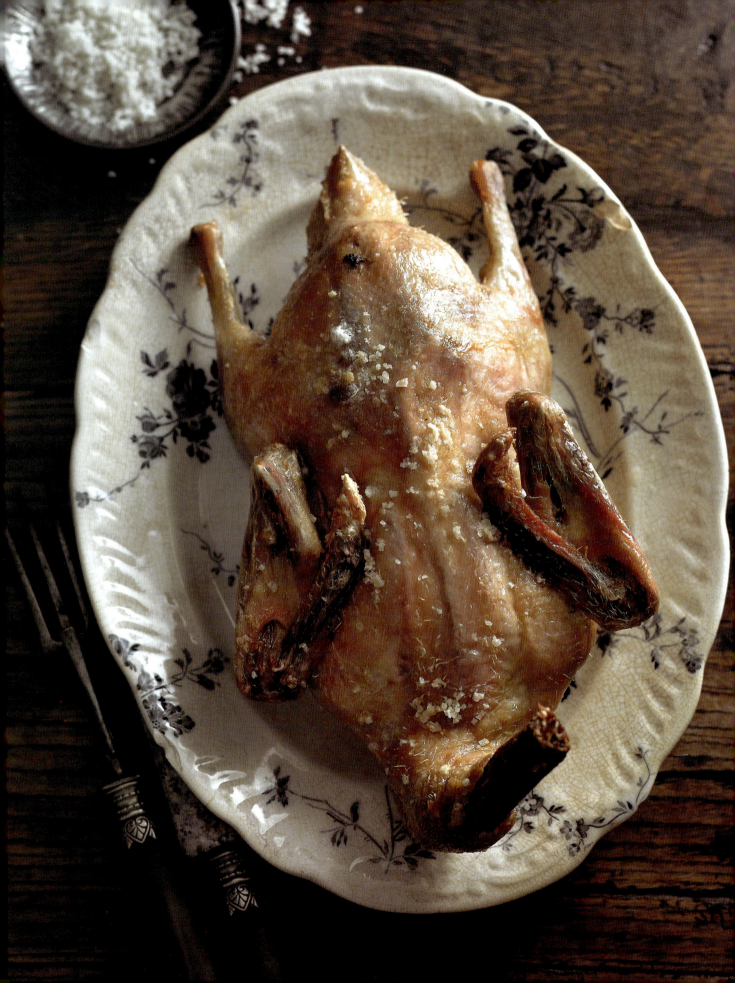

Duck is one of my favourite meats because I love collecting duck fat! It is a very stable fat for cooking, much like butter and coconut oil. There isn't as much meat on a duck as there is on a chicken but the flavour is far more intense. I pull off the meat and make a sweet, tangy duck salad (see page 162) or serve the breast with roast vegetables and keep the bones to make a potent Asian base stock. I want a free-roaming duck that had access to natural surroundings, sun, fresh air and water, just as I do with chickens. This imparts healthy nutrition and a good source of protein, and sits more comfortably with my ethics.

Ducks raised in a healthy manner impart healthy saturated fats. Saturated fats play many important roles in the body: they make up our cell membranes, strengthen the immune system, help suppress inflammation, and are involved in kidney function and hormone production. Saturated fats are required for the nervous system to function properly, and did you know that over half the fat in the brain is saturated? Saturated fats also carry the vital fat-soluble vitamins A, D and K2.

Roast duck

Serves 4–6 **PREP TIME:** *5 minutes* **COOKING TIME:** *3–3½ hours, depending on the size of the duck*

1 free-range duck
natural salt

1. Preheat the oven to 220°C (fan-forced).

2. Wash the duck under running water and pat dry with paper towels. Rub salt all over the duck, inside and out.

3. Place the duck in a roasting tin, breast-side down. Reduce the oven temperature to 120°C and roast until the duck is golden brown on the top. The roasting time depends on the size of the duck: smaller ducks up to 2 kg will need about 2¼ hours, but increase this to 2¾ hours for ducks weighing 2.5–3 kg.

4. Turn the duck over and put it back in the oven for 20 minutes or until the skin is golden brown. To check whether the duck is cooked through, pierce the thickest part with a large fork. If the fluid runs clear, the duck is cooked. If it is still pink, cook for another 15 minutes and check again.

5. Remove the duck from the oven and drain the fat into a glass jar. Store it in the fridge and use it for roasting vegetables and chicken, or pan-frying meat or eggs.

6. Pull off the duck meat to serve with your choice of vegetables or make a delicious duck salad (see page 162).

The first time I made this soup I was astounded by the flavour I created. It was a savoury taste known as umami, which can be described as a pleasant brothy or meaty taste with a long-lasting, mouthwatering and coating sensation over the tongue. Keep the duck bones from the roast duck on the previous page to make this delicious Asian-inspired soup.

Oriental duck soup

Serves 4 **PREP TIME:** *10 minutes* **COOKING TIME:** *1 hour 15 minutes*

reserved duck bones from a roast duck (see page 159)
natural salt
splash of apple cider vinegar
1 teaspoon Oriental Herb & Spice Blend or ground star anise, cardamom, cinnamon and garlic, to taste
2 carrots, thinly sliced
2 celery stalks and leaves, thinly sliced
3 spring onions, thinly sliced
2 cups (130 g) finely chopped kale
leftover roast duck meat (see page 159), shredded, to serve (optional)

1. Place the bones in a large saucepan with about 2 litres salted water and add the apple cider vinegar to help the bones break down and yield their mineral nutrients. Simmer over low–medium heat for 1 hour.

2. Drain the liquid, discarding the bones, then return the liquid to the pan and add the spice blend, carrot, celery, spring onion and kale. Simmer for 15 minutes or until the vegetables are cooked. If you like, add some shredded duck meat to each bowl, then ladle in the s oup and serve.

TIP: Store the bones in an airtight container in the freezer if you want to make the soup at a later date.

This is another way to eat roast duck meat. These delicious bite-sized morsels have a wonderful fresh flavour and are so simple to make – add them to a smorgasbord of finger food to share with friends.

Duck and grapefruit lettuce wraps

Serves 4 **PREP TIME:** *15 minutes*

leftover duck meat (see page 159), finely chopped
2 golden shallots, sliced
1 Lebanese cucumber, diced
1 grapefruit, segmented
1 large handful of coriander leaves, finely chopped
lime or grapefruit juice, to taste
sliced chilli (optional)
natural salt and freshly cracked pepper
8 large crispy lettuce leaves

1. Combine all the ingredients (except the lettuce leaves) in a bowl. Taste and adjust the seasoning, citrus juice or chilli to your liking. Spoon into the lettuce leaves, then wrap to enclose the filling and serve.

Pull the duck meat from your roast duck (see page 159) to use in this salad. The sweet and sour taste from the orange and pomegranate perfectly complements the savoury umami flavour of the duck, although mandarin or ruby grapefruit segments may be used instead of orange if preferred. Eat this salad with a cup or bowl of Oriental duck soup (see page 160).

Roast duck, cucumber, orange and pomegranate salad

Serves 4 **PREP TIME:** *15 minutes*

leftover roast duck meat and skin (see page 159), shredded
1 Lebanese cucumber, roughly chopped
1 orange, segmented
½ cup (125 ml) pomegranate seeds
2 spring onions, sliced
large handful of coriander or mint leaves
juice of 1 orange
natural salt and freshly cracked pepper

1. Place the duck meat and skin in a bowl. Add the cucumber, orange segments, pomegranate seeds, spring onion and coriander or mint.

2. Make a dressing by seasoning the orange juice with plenty of salt and pepper. Pour over the salad and gently toss to combine, then serve.

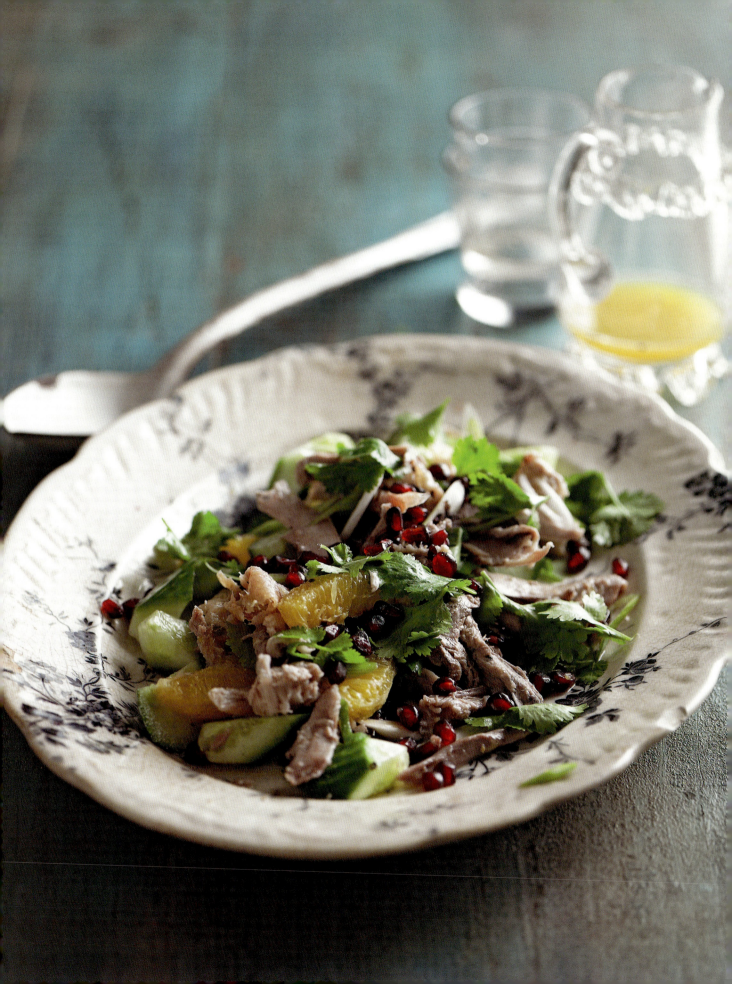

These bite-sized meatballs are dangerously moreish, and can be served in so many ways. Enjoy them simply with finely chopped flat-leaf parsley and lemon wedges, or with dips; add them to lunch boxes or finger food plates; wrap them in lettuce with a dip or dressing; or just serve them as they are with salad or vegetables. In cooler weather, when comfort food is called for, bake the meatballs in homemade tomato sauce (see page 227) with a scattering of parmesan cheese over the top.

Sweet onion meatballs

Serves 2–4   **PREP TIME:** *15 minutes*   **COOKING TIME:** *20 minutes*

---

65 g butter
1 onion, finely chopped
1 teaspoon Tuscan Herb & Spice Blend
    or dried oregano, basil and marjoram,
    to taste
natural salt
400 g minced beef, chicken, lamb, pork
    or a mixture of beef and pork
2 egg yolks
3 tablespoons olive oil
chopped flat-leaf parsley,
    to garnish (optional)

1. Melt half the butter in a frying pan over low heat, add the onion and cook, stirring, for 5 minutes or until transparent. Season with the spice blend and salt.

2. Transfer the onion mixture to a bowl, reserving the pan, then add the mince and egg yolks and mix well with your hands. Shape the mixture into 12 balls.

3. Heat the olive oil and remaining butter in the same frying pan over medium heat. Add the meatballs and cook, turning frequently, for 15 minutes or until cooked through and golden brown. Garnish with chopped parsley, if liked.

4. Alternatively, you may wish to bake the meatballs. Preheat the oven to 220°C (fan-forced) and grease a baking dish with butter and olive oil. Place the meatballs in the dish and reduce the oven temperature to 120°C. Bake for 30 minutes or until cooked through.

TIPS: You can replace the onion with leeks or golden shallots, if preferred. If you are making Indian-flavoured meatballs, replace the butter with ghee.

You can use other spice blends, if preferred: try Indian (or a curry leaf and ground cumin, turmeric and fenugreek, to taste) or Mexican (or sweet paprika and cayenne pepper, to taste).

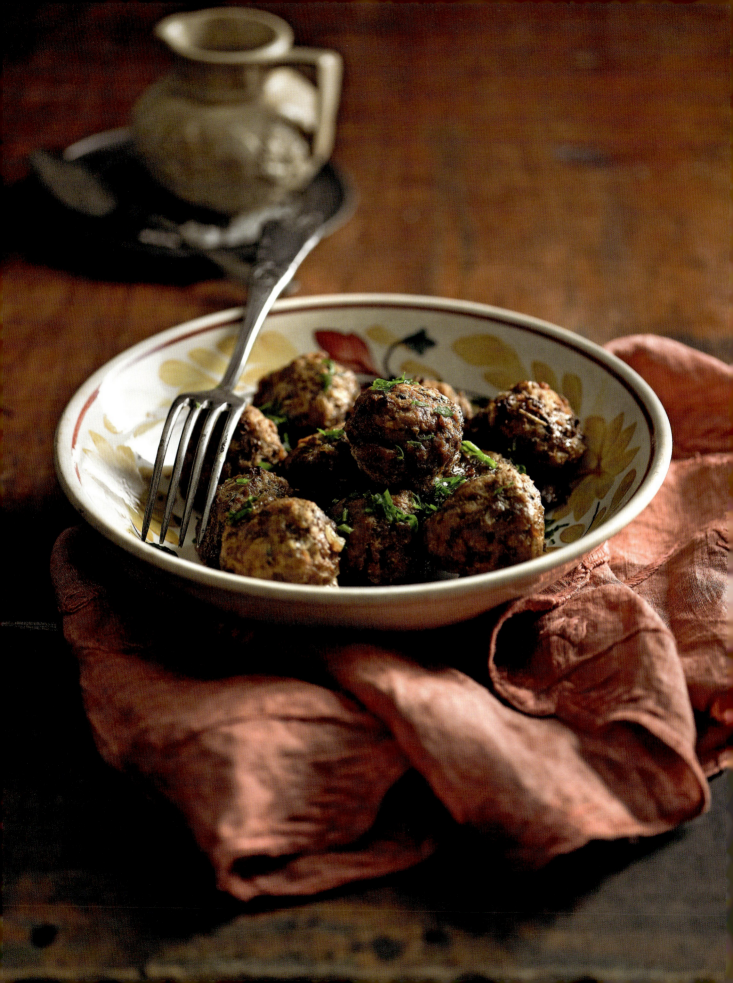

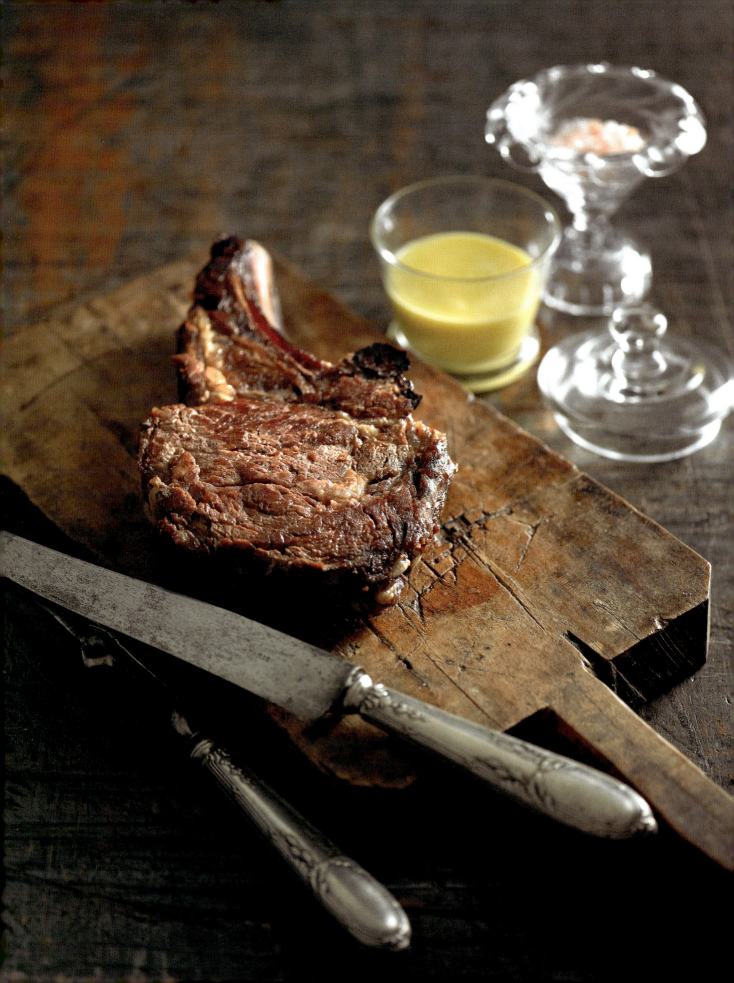

Searing a steak

One of the few times I turn my stove top up to high heat is when I am cooking a steak. It is very important to heat the pan well before adding the steak as this seals the surface, trapping in the juices. I am not a fan of non-stick cookware and rather than oiling the pan, I brush the steak with butter before cooking to prevent it from sticking to the pan.

Rare, medium or well done?

It very much depends on the thickness of the steak but there are a few guidelines I follow.

For rare, cook the steak for 2 minutes each side. Turn the steak only once, otherwise it will dry out. Always use tongs to handle steak as they won't pierce the meat, allowing the juices to escape. To test if your steak is done, press the centre with the back of the tongs. The steak will feel soft if it's rare.

To cook a steak medium or well done, place the seared rare steak in a baking dish and continue to cook in a preheated 120°C (fan-forced) oven. Press the back of the steak with tongs: if it is slightly firmer and springy it is medium, and if very firm it is well done. I don't give approximate times here as it varies so much, depending on the heat source and the thickness of the steak – cooking by feel is by far the most reliable guide.

Before serving, transfer the cooked steak to a plate, cover with baking paper and set aside to rest for 3–5 minutes. This allows the juices to settle and the muscle fibres to relax, which ensures the steak is tender. Season with freshly cracked pepper, natural salt and a squeeze of lemon juice or, to add heat and spice, add a sprinkling of Mexican Herb & Spice Blend (or sweet paprika and cayenne pepper, to taste). Serve with vegetables or salad and your favourite dip (see page 98).

See page 29 for information on the detrimental effects of high-temperature cooking.

I have very happy memories of enjoying chops and cutlets as a child. My brother and I used to argue over how many we had on our plates and fight for more! This simple recipe is my mother's. I've always adored the taste of lamb fat infused with salt and lemon, and suspect this might be where my love for chewing on bones began. Just like grass-fed beef, lamb is a rich source of protein, B vitamins, vitamin D, iron, zinc and omega-3 essential fats. The cutlets are delicious served with Smooth cauliflower mash and Tabouli sans grain (see pages 111 and 118).

Pan-fried lamb cutlets

Serves 2 **PREP TIME:** *5 minutes* **COOKING TIME:** *10 minutes*

40 g butter
2 tablespoons olive oil
8 lamb cutlets
natural salt and freshly cracked pepper
juice of 1 lemon

1. Melt the butter and olive oil in a frying pan over medium heat, add the cutlets and season with salt and pepper. Cook for 5 minutes, then turn them over and cook for another 5 minutes. Remove to a plate, then cover with foil and leave to rest for 2 minutes or so. Serve with the lemon juice and more salt, to taste.

The sweet spices of star anise, cinnamon and clove combined with apple and pork are a culinary match made in heaven. Making good crackle is easy and the extra preparation time is worth it!

Roast pork belly with apple, cabbage and fennel

Serves 4–6 **PREP TIME:** *15 minutes, plus chilling time* **COOKING TIME:** *about 4 hours*

1.5 kg pork belly
1 teaspoon natural salt
2 tablespoons Oriental Herb & Spice Blend or ground star anise, cardamom, cinnamon and garlic, to taste
2 green apples, sliced
1 cup (80 g) shredded white cabbage
2 small fennel bulbs, sliced
1 cup (250 ml) bone stock (see page 214) or water

1. Place the pork belly, skin-side up, on a wire rack over the sink. Pour boiling water over the pork skin – this will help the skin crisp up into crunchy crackling. Pat the pork completely dry with paper towel and place, uncovered, in the refrigerator for 2 hours.

2. Preheat the oven to its highest temperature.

3. Remove the pork from the fridge and place, skin-side up, on a chopping board. Using a very sharp knife, score the pork belly skin deeply (without cutting into the meat). Grind the salt and spice blend in a mortar and pestle and rub into the scored skin.

4. Place the apple, cabbage, fennel and stock or water in a roasting tin and sprinkle with salt. Place the pork belly on the vegetables, scored-side up. Reduce the oven temperature to 120°C and roast for 3–4 hours or until the skin has crackled beautifully and the meat is well cooked and soft. Check the base of the dish during cooking to ensure it doesn't dry out – add extra water as needed.

5. Remove the pork belly and rest on a board for 5 minutes, then carve and serve with the succulent apple, fennel and cabbage.

These wonderfully succulent lamb chops simply melt in your mouth. The fresh herbs cut through the fat, making them easier to digest. To make the most of the flavours in the herb paste, prepare the chops the night before you want to eat them so they have plenty of time to marinate.

Marinated lamb chops

Serves 2 **PREP TIME:** *5 minutes, plus marinating time* **COOKING TIME:** *30 minutes*

½ teaspoon coarse natural salt, plus extra to serve
½ teaspoon whole black peppercorns
2 cloves garlic, peeled
handful of mint leaves
handful of flat-leaf parsley leaves
3 tablespoons olive oil
4 lamb chops
½ lemon, sliced
lemon juice, to serve
Tomato with fresh curd and cucumber ribbons salad (see page 115), to serve (optional)

1. Place the salt, peppercorns, garlic, mint, parsley and olive oil in a mortar and pestle and pound to a paste. Rub the paste over the chops, then place in a baking dish with a few lemon slices. Cover and refrigerate overnight.

2. Preheat the oven to 200°C (fan-forced). Take the chops out of the fridge 15 minutes before baking.

3. Reduce the oven temperature to 120°C and bake the chops for 30 minutes or until golden brown and cooked to your liking. Serve with extra salt, lots of lemon juice and the tomato salad, if liked.

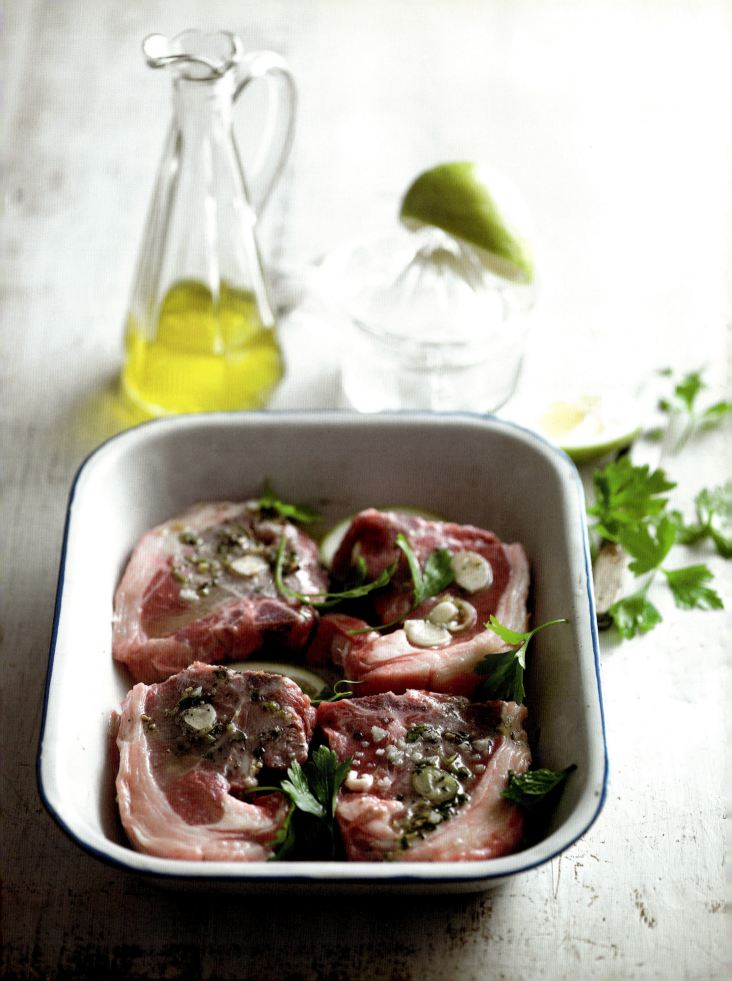

This dish is perfect for cheaper or less fashionable cuts of meat because slow cooking effortlessly tenderises the meat. If you have a slow cooker you can use that instead and cook it on low for 8 hours. It is quite a dry curry, but the coconut and pumpkin sweeten the meat and the spices give it a warm infusion.

Slow-cooked spicy beef and coconut pumpkin curry

Serves 4–6 **PREP TIME:** *25 minutes* **COOKING TIME:** *8 hours*

⅓ cup (80 ml) coconut oil
2 brown onions, diced
2 celery stalks, sliced
3 tablespoons Indian Herb & Spice Blend or a curry leaf and ground cumin, turmeric and fenugreek, to taste
1 kg chuck steak, cut into 2 cm cubes
½ pumpkin (squash), thickly sliced
1 young coconut, flesh and water scooped out and pureed
natural salt
Steamed greens and Minty cucumber yoghurt dip (see pages 103 and 98), to serve
coriander leaves, to garnish (optional)

1. Preheat the oven to 120°C (fan-forced).

2. Heat the coconut oil in a cast-iron casserole dish over medium heat, add the onion, celery and spice blend and saute for 5 minutes or until the onion is transparent. Add the meat and cook until browned but not cooked through.

3. Add the pumpkin, coconut puree, 1 cup (250 ml) water and season well with salt. Stir to combine, then cover and cook in the oven for 6–8 hours.

4. Serve with steamed greens, cucumber yoghurt dip and a scattering of coriander leaves, if liked.

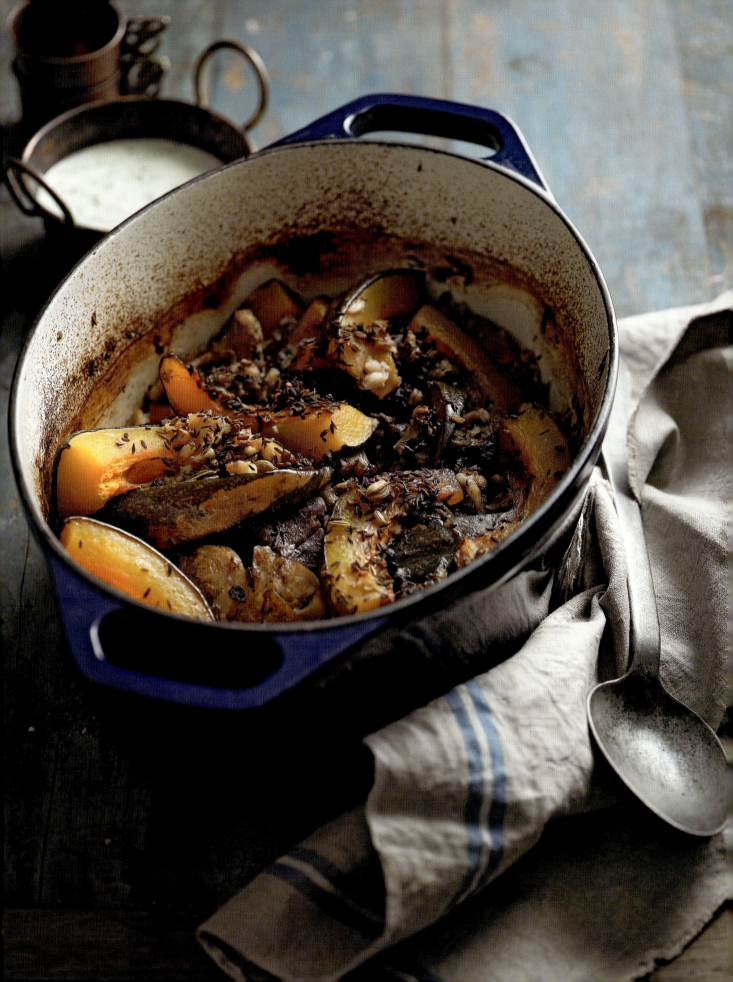

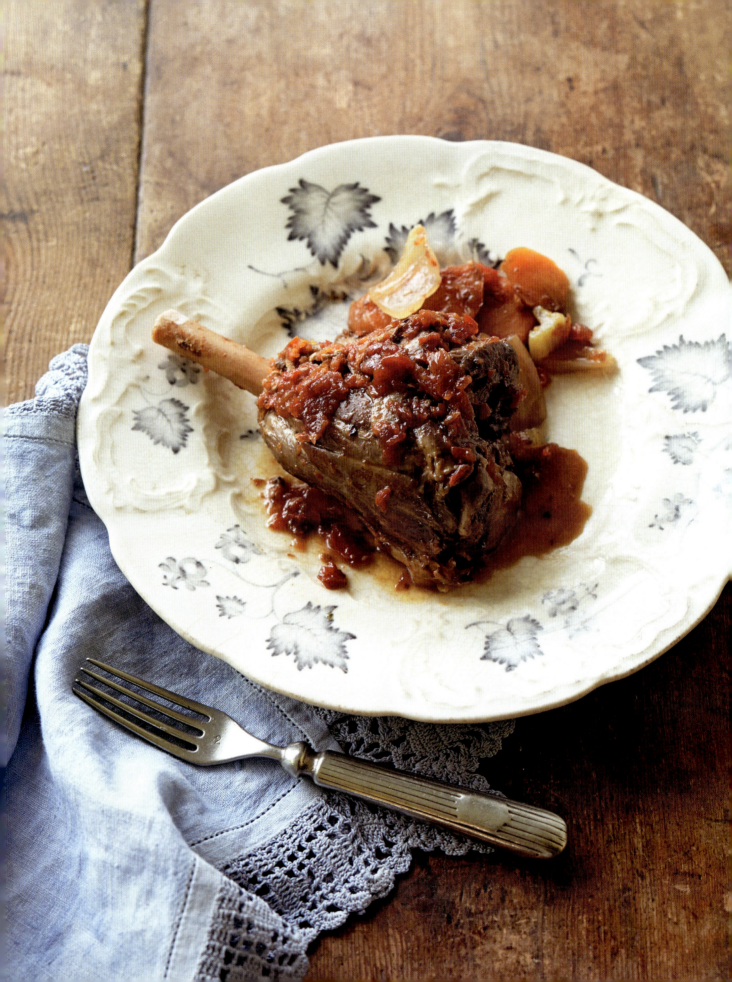

This is one meal I love to enjoy on my own so I can chew the bone and suck out the bone marrow to complete my meal. This might not be very ladylike but who's watching? It's just too good . . . Serve with a simple salad, such as Leafy greens and herb salad on page 115.

Slow-cooked Tuscan lamb shanks

Serves 6 **PREP TIME:** *20 minutes* **COOKING TIME:** *8 hours*

4 carrots, thickly sliced
4 celery stalks, with leaf tops, thickly sliced
12 tomatoes, chopped
1 large brown onion, diced
4 cloves garlic, sliced
2 bay leaves
2 cups (500 ml) beef bone stock (see page 214) or water
natural salt and freshly cracked pepper
2 tablespoons Tuscan Herb & Spice Blend or dried oregano, basil and marjoram, to taste
80 g butter
6 lamb shanks, french-trimmed

1. Arrange the carrot, celery, tomato, onion and garlic in layers in the slow cooker. Add the bay leaves and stock or water, and season with salt, pepper and the spice blend. Rub butter over the lamb shanks, then nestle the shanks in the vegetables. Cover and cook on low for 8 hours.

VARIATION
Osso buco cooks beautifully in a slow cooker or cast-iron casserole dish. Heat equal quantities of butter and olive oil in a frying pan or casserole dish and saute 2 cross-cut veal shanks per person in a mixture of chopped tomato, carrot, onion, celery and garlic, as well as aromatics such as a cinnamon quill, bay leaf or juniper berries. Transfer all the ingredients to your slow cooker (or leave in the casserole dish) and pour in with enough beef stock or water to half cover. Cover and cook on low for 8 hours (or if using a casserole, in a preheated 120°C (fan-forced) oven for 6–8 hours). I love to serve this with sweet potato mash and steamed spinach (see pages 111 and 103).

The melt-in-your-mouth, golden fat that is naturally released when these ribs are slow-cooked is a delicious consequence of healthy grass-fed animals. Try them once and you'll never go back. See pages 14 and 16 for more information about grass-feeding.

Beef short ribs with Sunday Roast Blend

Serves 6   **PREP TIME:** *10 minutes*   **COOKING TIME:** *4 hours*

1 kg chopped beef short ribs
2 onions, chopped
natural salt
3 tablespoons Sunday Roast Blend or dried rosemary, thyme, sage and oregano, to taste
finely grated zest and juice of 2 lemons
cultured vegetables (see page 221) and steamed greens, to serve

1. Preheat the oven to 200°C (fan-forced).

2. Place the ribs and onion in a large roasting tin, season with salt and the Sunday Roast Blend. Cover with baking paper and foil, then reduce the oven temperature to 120°C and roast for 4 hours. (If preferred, you can cook the ribs in a slow cooker on low heat for 6–8 hours.) Scatter over the lemon zest and juice and serve with cultured vegetables and steamed greens.

TIP: To add extra heat, add a little Spanish Hot Blend or sweet paprika and cayenne pepper, to taste.

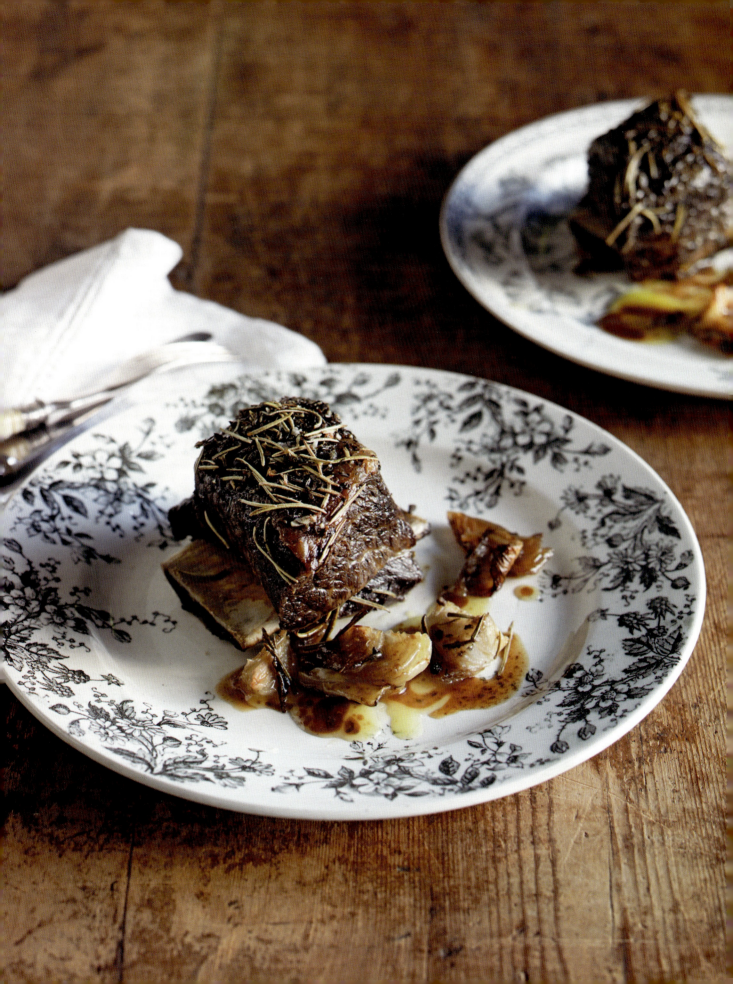

Long, slow cooking results in crisp, succulent chicken that falls off the bone. Chew all the cartilage between the joints and eat the giblets for extra nutrition.

Roast chicken

Serves 4–6 **PREP TIME:** *15 minutes* **COOKING TIME:** *about 3 hours*

2 tomatoes, cut into quarters
2 leeks, thickly sliced or 1 large onion, cut into quarters
2 carrots, thickly sliced
2 celery stalks, thickly sliced
1 bulb garlic
1.5 kg chicken
½ lemon
2 tablespoons duck fat or olive oil
natural salt
40 g butter, softened
1–2 tablespoons Provincial Herb & Spice Blend or dried rosemary, thyme and sage, to taste
3 tablespoons finely chopped flat-leaf parsley (optional)
Leafy greens and herb salad (see page 115), to serve

Gravy
80 g butter
juice of ½ lemon
natural salt and freshly cracked pepper

1. Preheat the oven to 220°C (fan-forced). Place all the vegetables in a baking dish or roasting tin and roughly toss to combine.

2. Wash the chicken inside and out and pat dry with paper towel, then rub lemon all over the skin, followed by the duck fat or olive oil. Rub some salt in the cavity. Gently spread the butter between the skin and breast meat and massage it in, taking care not to tear the skin. Place the chicken on the vegetables, breast-side up or down, and sprinkle with the spice blend.

3. Reduce the oven temperature to 120°C and roast for about 2 hours or until the chicken is golden brown. Remove from the oven and baste well with all the lovely juices. Turn the chicken over and put it back in the oven for another hour or so, to achieve golden brown skin on the other side. Check that the chicken is cooked by piercing the thickest part with a large fork – the juices should run clear. If they are still a bit pink, cook for another 15 minutes and check again.

4. Transfer the chicken and vegetables (except the garlic) to a platter and cover with baking paper and foil to keep warm.

5. To make the gravy, pour the pan juices into a small saucepan. Squeeze the soft flesh from the garlic cloves into the pan, discarding the skins. Bring the gravy to a simmer, then strain into a clean saucepan and stir in the butter and lemon juice. Taste and season if needed.

6. Pour the gravy over the chicken. Sprinkle with chopped parsley, if liked, and serve with the roast vegetables and salad.

STUFFING!
This is my recipe using an organic stuffing blend we make at Ovvio. Finely dice a red onion and gently saute in 60 g butter or 3 tablespoons olive oil until soft and transparent. Tip into a bowl, along with the excess butter or oil, and mix with 1 cup (100 g) Roast Chicken Stuffing Blend (a mixture of breadcrumbs, sage, thyme and garlic). Remove the skin from 400 g pork or chicken sausages and add to the bowl. Mix well with your hands, then stuff into the chicken cavity before roasting.

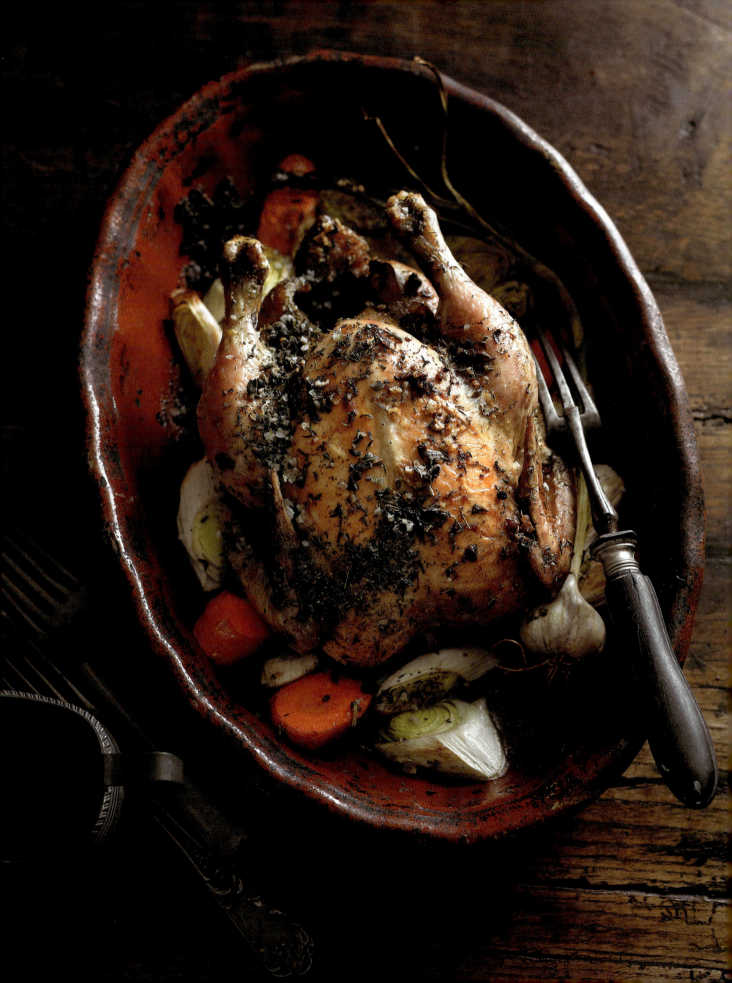

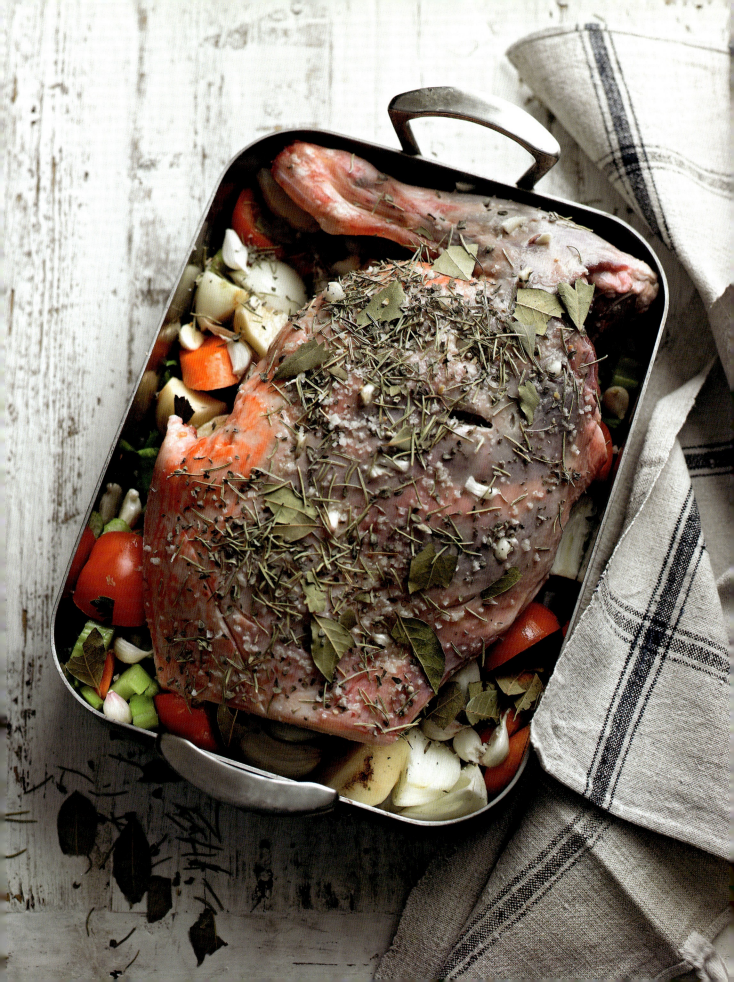

This much-loved dish is traditionally served on a Sunday with roast potatoes and carrots, green vegetables and gravy. And it keeps on giving – the leftovers are fantastic in salads and sandwiches during the week.

Roast leg of lamb

Serves 4–6 **PREP TIME:** *15 minutes* **COOKING TIME:** *about 4 hours*

2 tomatoes, cut into quarters
4 potatoes, cut into quarters
2 onions, cut into quarters
2 carrots, thickly sliced
2 celery stalks, sliced
1 cup (250 ml) bone stock (see page 214) or water
natural salt
2 kg leg of lamb or shoulder
2 tablespoons olive oil
40 g butter
4 cloves garlic, cut into quarters lengthways
2 tablespoons Grecian Herb & Spice Blend (or bay leaf, dried rosemary and oregano and black pepper, to taste) or Sunday Roast Blend (or dried rosemary, thyme, sage and oregano, to taste)
steamed greens (see page 103), to serve

1. Preheat the oven to 220°C (fan-forced). Place the vegetables in a roasting tin and roughly toss to combine. Pour over the stock or water and season with salt.

2. Rub the lamb with the olive oil, butter and some salt. Pierce the lamb with a sharp knife 16 times and put the garlic quarters in the slits.

3. Place the lamb on the vegetables then scatter over the spice blend. Cover with baking paper and foil.

4. Reduce the oven temperature to 120°C and roast for about 4 hours or until the lamb is cooked through and falling off the bone. Baste well during the cooking time. For the last 15–20 minutes, remove the paper and foil and turn the temperature up so the meat browns nicely.

5. Take it out of the oven and let it rest, covered, for about 15 minutes before serving. Carve and serve with the roast vegetables and steamed greens. If you want to make a gravy, follow the instructions for roast chicken gravy on page 178 but use the pan juices from the roast lamb.

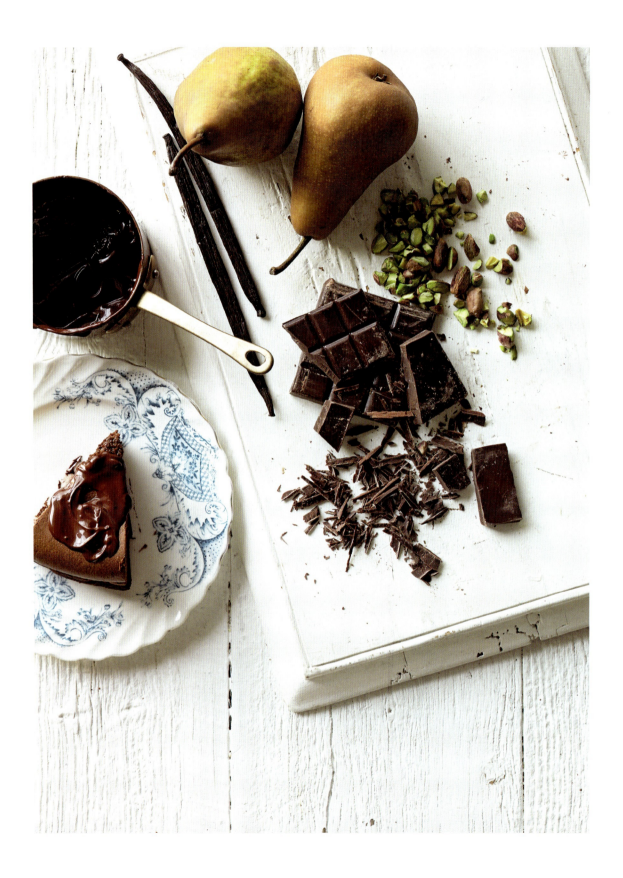

Desserts

The following desserts are not based on any particular tradition or culture but were created to offer a grain-free, sugar-free alternative to modern, sugar-dense and highly processed types. They are for special occasions, just as sweet foods were for ancient civilisations. Through the medieval period, sugar was considered a fine spice and was used as a flavour enhancer in a similar fashion to cinnamon or nutmeg.

These delightful offerings are made with whole-food ingredients without any of the detrimental side-effects of sugar and are nutritionally good for you. I've created recipes for cakes, biscuits, macaroons, crumbles, mousse, wobbly jelly and popsicles, even old-fashioned candy jellies that are so satisfying that even a sugar addict will be content.

The cakes and macaroons are served daily at our Ovvio tea house with a pot of tea, enabling our clients and customers to recharge and enjoy a moment of stillness.

If sweet desserts don't take your fancy, enjoy a platter of fresh fruit and cheese just like the French. Choose your own way to finish the meal with something a little special.

These are so easy to make, but I warn you now: they are very moreish. You only need the egg whites for this recipe, so keep the egg yolks to make a mayonnaise or to add to a richly eggy omelette.

Coconut macaroons

Makes 16 **PREP TIME:** *15 minutes* **COOKING TIME:** *15 minutes*

9 egg whites
3 tablespoons coconut sugar or raw honey
¼ teaspoon vanilla bean powder
about 3 cups (240 g) desiccated coconut, plus extra for coating (optional)
spring or filtered water, or orange or rosewater (optional)

1. Preheat the oven to 200°C (fan-forced). Line a baking tray with baking paper.

2. Beat the egg whites, sugar or honey and vanilla until fluffy, then fold in enough desiccated coconut to bind (you may not need it all). If the mixture feels a bit dry, add a splash of spring, filtered or floral water to bind it. Roll the mixture into 16 balls, then roll to coat in extra coconut, if liked.

3. Reduce the oven temperature to 180°C. Place the balls on the prepared tray and bake for 10–15 minutes or until lightly golden. Allow to cool, then store in an airtight container in the fridge for up to 4 days.

VARIATIONS (pictured right)

Chocolate coconut macaroons: Add ⅓ cup (35 g) raw cocoa powder to the mixture.

Orange coconut macaroons: Stir in 2 teaspoons finely grated orange zest for added citrus zing. Decorate with small pieces of orange rind, if liked.

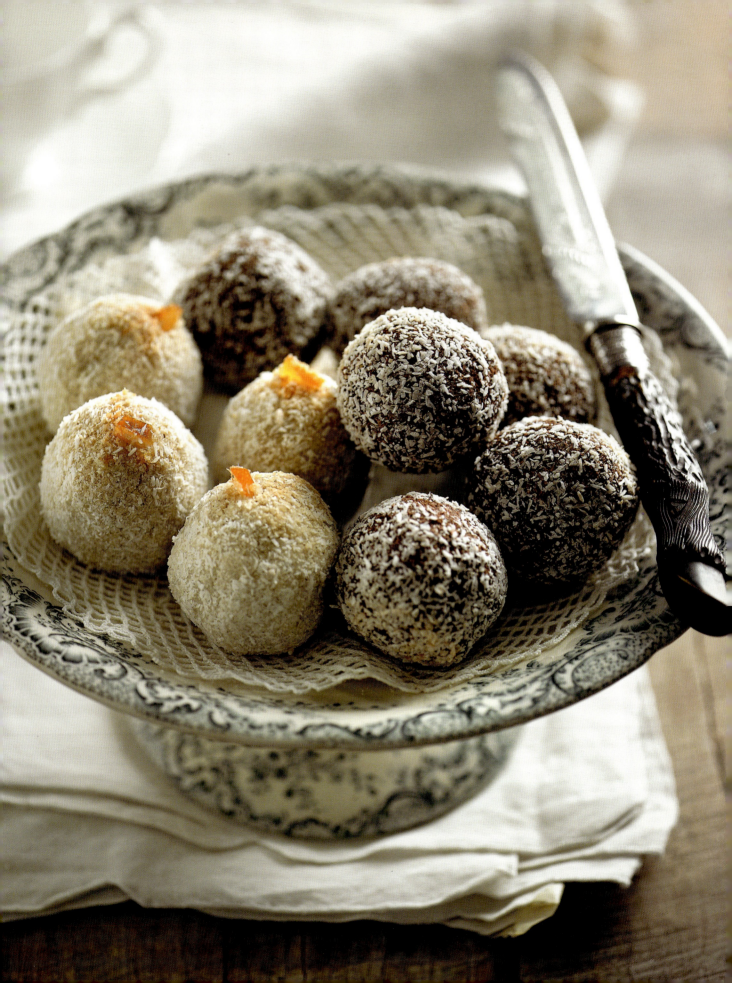

When I serve this to my friends, no one believes it is made without flour! But it's true and here is the recipe to prove it. It's light and moist with a wonderfully delicate flavour – a superior rival to any processed ready-to-go snack.

Vanilla pear almond cake

Serves 8   **PREP TIME:** *15 minutes*   **COOKING TIME:** *1 hour 15 minutes*

---

4 pears
6 eggs, separated
⅓ cup (75 g) coconut sugar
2 ½ cups (300 g) almond meal or ground activated almonds
1 teaspoon vanilla bean powder
pinch of natural salt
3 tablespoons almond flakes
cream or yoghurt (see page 218), to serve

1. Preheat the oven to 200°C (fan-forced). Line the base of a 20 cm springform cake tin with baking paper and oil the side with coconut oil.

2. Peel and roughly chop the pears and place in a medium saucepan with 1 cup (250 ml) water. Cover and bring to a simmer over medium heat, then poach for 10–15 minutes. Drain, reserving the pear water to make jelly, if liked (see page 202). Set aside to cool.

3. While the pears are cooling, beat the egg whites until stiff peaks form.

4. Transfer the pears to a food processor and puree until smooth. Add the egg yolks and coconut sugar and beat until creamy. Add the almond meal or ground almonds, vanilla and salt and process until combined. Gently fold the egg white into the pear mixture, keeping as much lightness and air in the mixture as you can. The purpose of folding is to retain the air you have beaten into the whites – use a light touch, and never use an electric mixer for this step. Pour into the prepared cake tin.

5. Reduce the oven temperature to 180°C and bake for 1 hour or until a skewer inserted in the centre comes out clean. Place the tin on a wire rack to cool completely. Sprinkle the cake with the almond flakes and serve with cream or yoghurt.

6. The cake will keep in an airtight container in the fridge for up to 4 days.

VARIATIONS

Cinnamon apple almond cake
Replace the pears with 4 cooked and pureed apples. Add 1 teaspoon cinnamon powder instead of the vanilla.

Vanilla orange almond cake
Replace the pears with 2 unwaxed oranges. Place the whole oranges (with skin) in a medium saucepan with 1 cup (250 ml) water and simmer, covered, for 10 minutes or until soft. Drain, then puree the oranges and allow to cool. Proceed with the recipe.

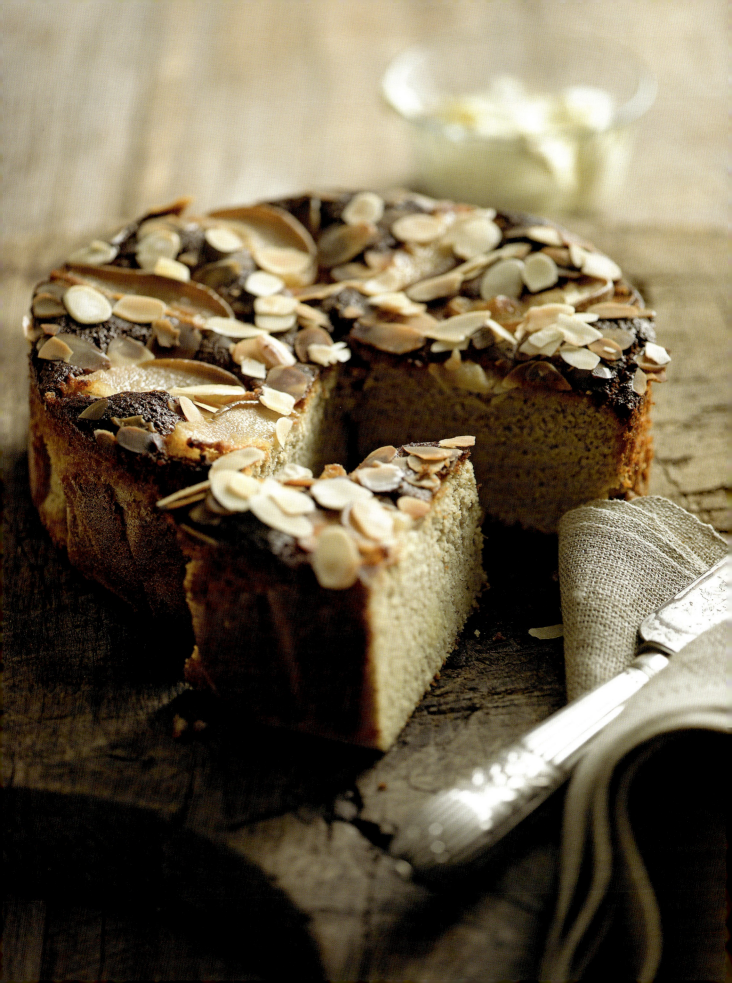

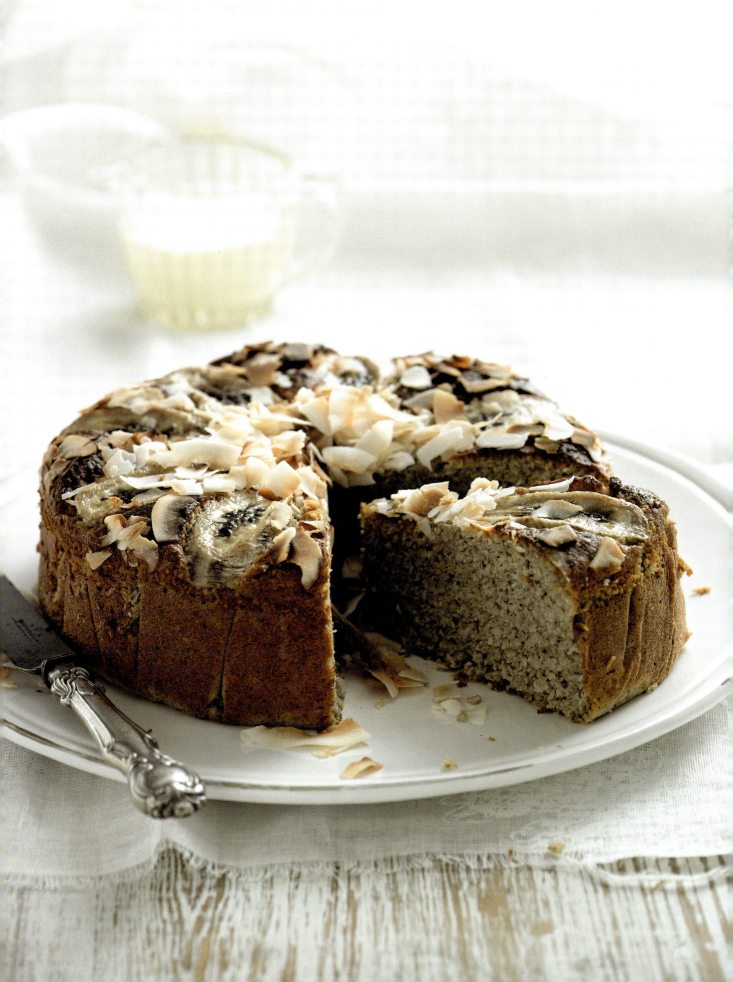

This cake puts a smile on kids' faces – and adults' too! It is happiness on a plate and goodness for your health. Serve it with cream or yoghurt.

Vanilla banana coconut cake

Serves 8 **PREP TIME:** *15 minutes* **COOKING TIME:** *1 hour*

6 eggs, separated
⅓ cup (75 g) coconut sugar
5 ripe bananas
2 ½ cups (200 g) desiccated coconut
1 teaspoon vanilla bean powder
pinch of natural salt
3 tablespoons coarsely shredded coconut
cream or yoghurt (see page 218), to serve

1. Preheat the oven to 200°C (fan-forced). Line the base of a 20 cm springform cake tin with baking paper and oil the side with coconut oil.

2. In a bowl beat the egg whites until stiff peaks form.

Place the egg yolks and coconut sugar in a food processor and beat until creamy. Add the bananas and process, and then the desiccated coconut, vanilla and salt and process until combined. Gently fold the banana mixture into the egg whites, keeping as much lightness and air in the mixture as you can. The purpose of folding is to retain the air you have beaten into the whites – use a light touch, and never use an electric mixer for this step. Pour into the prepared tin.

3. Reduce the oven temperature to 180°C and bake for 1 hour or until a skewer inserted in the centre comes out clean. Place the tin on a wire rack to cool completely. Sprinkle the cake with the shredded coconut and serve with cream or yoghurt.

4. The cake will keep in an airtight container in the fridge for up to 4 days.

TIP: If you don't have a food processor, you can use an electric mixer instead. Just make sure you mash the bananas well first.

VARIATIONS

Cinnamon pear coconut cake
Replace the mashed banana with 4 cooked and pureed pears. Add 1 teaspoon cinnamon powder instead of the vanilla.

Spiced apple coconut cake
Replace the mashed banana with 4 cooked and pureed apples. Instead of the vanilla, add 1 teaspoon All Things Nice Blend or ground cinnamon, cloves and nutmeg, to taste.

This is the most popular cake at Ovvio. We serve it with thick organic cream and a pot of organic tea. Like a cloud, it's light and airy – there's hardly anything in it – but it is wonderfully chocolatey.

Chocolate cloud cake

Serves 8 **PREP TIME:** *20 minutes* **COOKING TIME:** *35 minutes*

350 g dark chocolate, broken into pieces
50 g butter
2 tablespoons raw honey (optional)
10 eggs, separated
½ teaspoon vanilla bean powder
thick cream, to serve (optional)

1. Preheat the oven to 180°C (fan-forced). Line the base of a 20 cm springform cake tin with baking paper and oil the side with coconut oil.

2. First melt the chocolate and butter. Quarter fill a saucepan with water and heat until simmering. Place the chocolate pieces and butter in a heatproof bowl, then set the bowl over the simmering water, but do not allow the base of the bowl to touch the water or any water to get into the bowl. Stir until the chocolate and butter have melted. Stir in the honey (if using) and set aside to cool slightly.

3. In a bowl beat the egg whites until stiff peaks form.

4. Place the egg yolks and vanilla in another bowl and blend well. Slowly add the melted chocolate mixture and mix until just combined (make sure it is not hot as you don't want to cook the eggs). Gently fold in one third of the egg whites, keeping as much lightness and air in the mixture as you can, then fold in the rest. The purpose of folding is to retain the air you have beaten into the whites – use a light touch, and never use an electric mixer for this step. Pour the batter into the prepared tin.

5. Reduce the oven temperature to 150°C and bake for 35 minutes or until a skewer inserted in the centre comes out clean. Place the tin on a wire rack to cool completely. Serve with a dollop of cream, if liked.

6. The cake will keep in an airtight container in the fridge for up to 4 days.

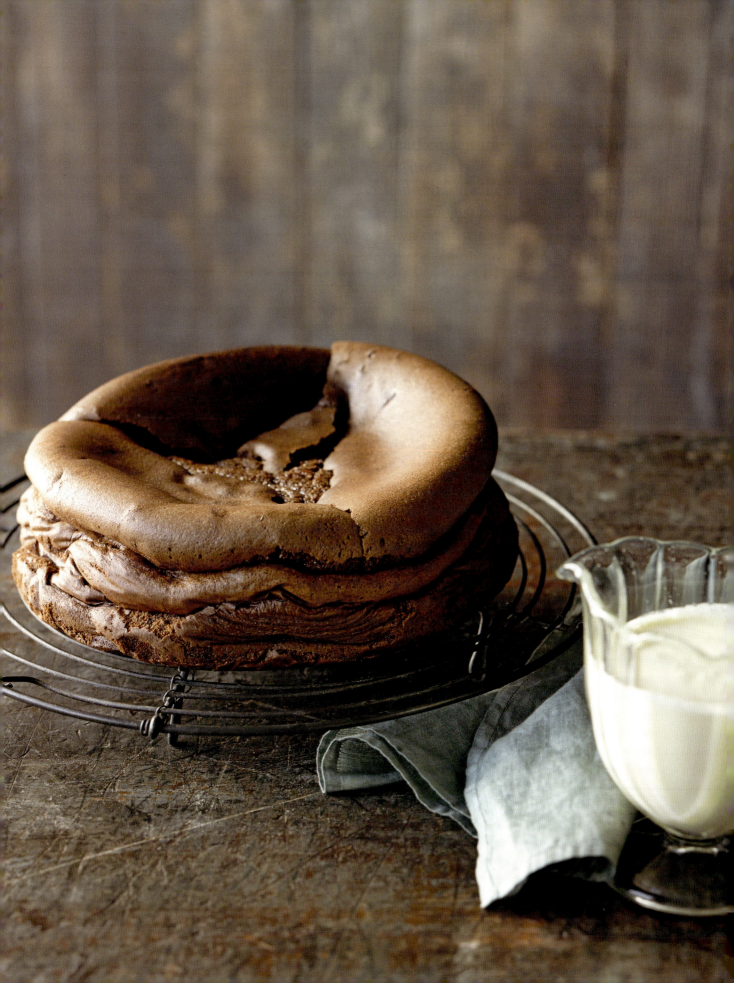

Delightful, delicious, delicate, satisfying and wholesome, this could possibly be one of my favourite cakes. Well . . . next to the Chocolate cloud cake on page 190. You can eat this for breakfast or as a snack on the run – it's a complete meal!

Zucchini and carrot cake with lemon vanilla cream-cheese icing

Serves 8 **PREP TIME:** 15 minutes **COOKING TIME:** 1 hour

4 eggs, separated
150 g raw honey
finely grated zest of 1 small lemon (reserve the juice for the icing)
150 g almond meal or ground activated almonds
1 carrot, grated
1 small zucchini (courgette), grated
½ teaspoon natural salt
fresh fruit, to serve (optional)

Lemon vanilla cream-cheese icing

juice of 1 small lemon
½ teaspoon vanilla bean powder
1 cup (200 g) fresh curd (see page 216) or store-bought Quark or ricotta cheese
1 tablespoon raw honey

1. Preheat the oven to 200°C (fan-forced). Line the base of a 20 cm springform cake tin with baking paper and oil the side with coconut oil.

2. In a bowl beat the egg whites until stiff peaks form.

3. Place the egg yolks in a second bowl, add the honey and beat until creamy. Add the lemon zest, almond meal or ground almonds, carrot, zucchini and salt and blend until combined. Gently fold in the egg white, then pour into the prepared cake tin.

4. Reduce the oven temperature to 180°C and bake for 1 hour or until a skewer inserted in the centre comes out clean. Place the tin on a wire rack to cool completely.

5. To make the icing, mix together all the ingredients in a bowl.

6. Spread the icing over the cooled cake and serve as is, or with fresh fruit. The cake will keep in an airtight container in the fridge for up to 4 days.

VARIATION

Double the quantities for the cake batter and make 2 cakes, sandwiched together with icing, for a decadent but healthy feast! This is what we did in the photo, but of course a single iced cake is just as delicious.

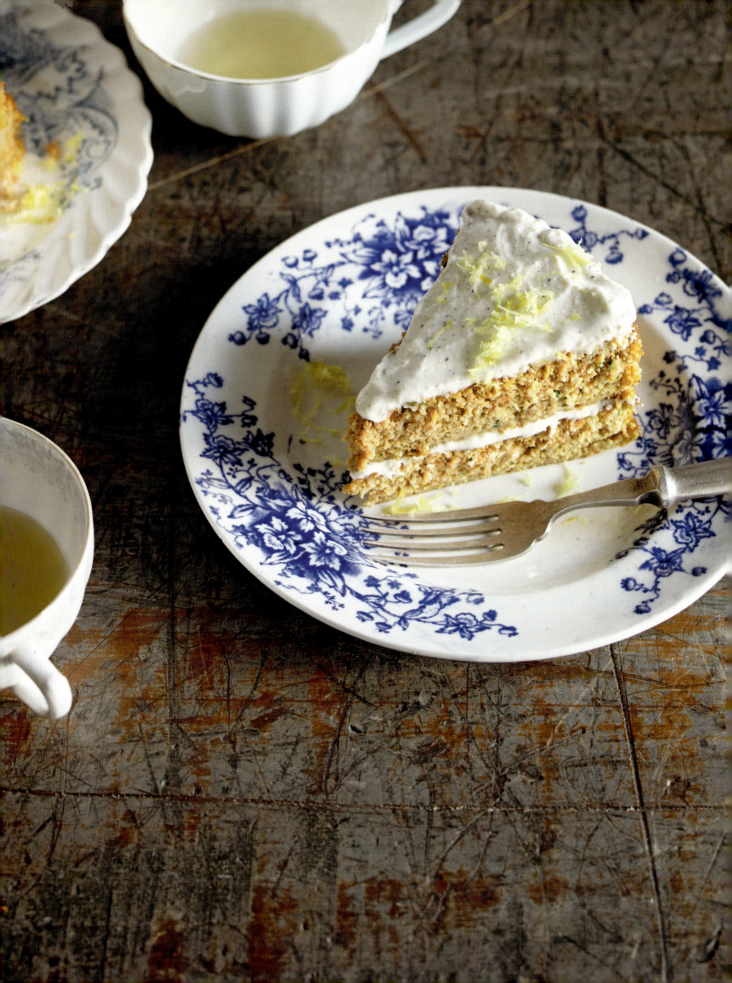

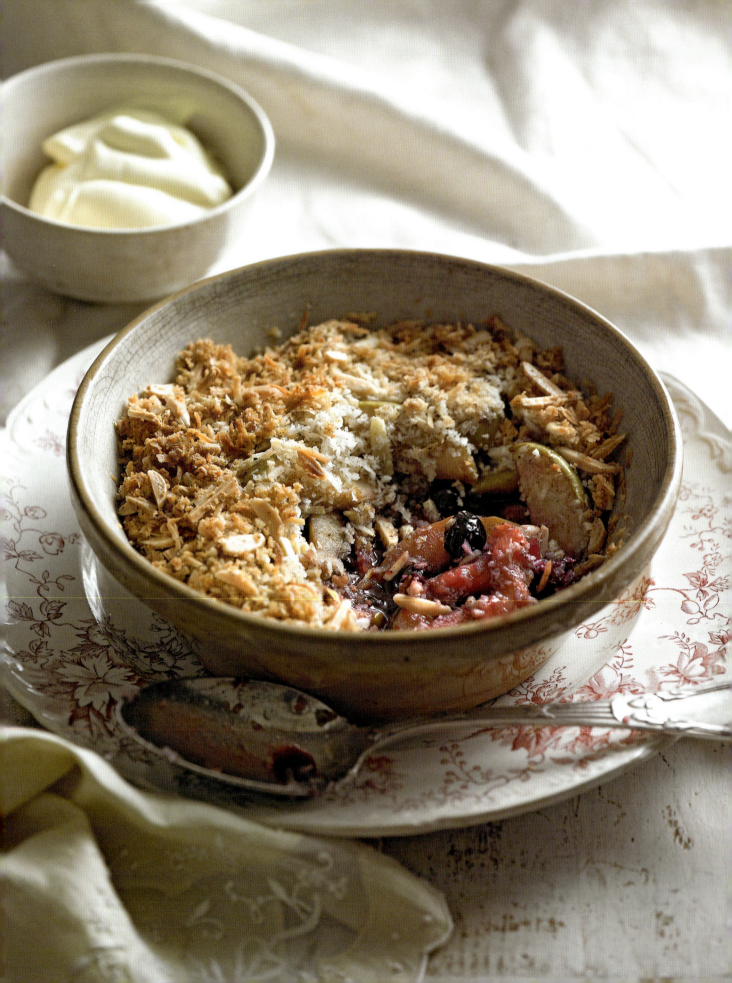

This crumble reminds me of autumn, the season of harvest and the fruition of growth during spring and summer. I've used blueberries and apples here but you can use any type of berry and other autumn fruit such as rhubarb, quince, pears and pomegranates. Follow the poached fruit recipe on page 199 to cook rhubarb and quince before using them in a crumble. Pears are like apples and are fine to go in raw. This is also great for breakfast!

Apple and blueberry crumble

Serves 4–6 **PREP TIME:** *15 minutes* **COOKING TIME:** *30 minutes*

---

3 medium green apples, cored (but leave the skin on) and sliced
1 cup (150 g) blueberries
½ teaspoon All Things Nice Spice Blend or ground cinnamon, cloves and nutmeg, to taste
1 tablespoon coconut sugar or ½ teaspoon stevia green leaf powder
cream or yoghurt (see page 218), to serve

Coconut crumble

1 cup (75 g) shredded coconut
½ cup (70 g) slivered almonds
½ teaspoon vanilla bean powder
3 tablespoons coconut oil

1. Preheat the oven to 180°C (fan-forced).

2. Combine the apple, berries, spice blend and sugar or stevia powder in a bowl. Pour into a shallow medium baking dish and add about ⅓ cup (80 ml) water.

3. To make the coconut crumble, place all the ingredients in a bowl and mix to combine.

4. Spread the crumble mixture over the fruit, then reduce the oven temperature to 160°C and bake for 30 minutes or until the top is golden brown and fruit is cooked. Serve with cream or yoghurt.

If you crave salty, savoury foods and can ravage a bag of crisps or crackers in one sitting, then this healthy alternative is not only good for you, but will also satisfy your cravings. Eat the biscuits just as they are or serve as part of a dessert cheese plate with cheese, fresh pear slices and pate (see page 228).

Parmesan biscuits

Makes about 18 **PREP TIME:** *15 minutes* **COOKING TIME:** *25 minutes*

2 cups (240 g) almond meal or ground activated almonds
2 teaspoons Tuscan Herb & Spice Blend (or dried oregano, basil and marjoram, to taste) or Mexican Herb & Spice Blend (or sweet paprika and cayenne pepper, to taste)
1 teaspoon fine natural salt
1 cup (80 g) very finely grated aged parmesan cheese
2 tablespoons extra virgin olive oil, more if needed
⅓ cup (80 ml) spring or filtered water, more if needed
1 egg white, lightly beaten

1. Preheat the oven to 200°C (fan-forced). Line a large baking tray with baking paper.

2. Place all the ingredients in a bowl and combine with your hands until a moist, moderately sticky dough forms (add more water or oil if you need it).

3. Using oiled hands, place the dough on the prepared tray and flatten with the palm of your hand. Press the dough out evenly until quite thin. If it cracks, simply press it back together with moist fingers.

4. Reduce the oven temperature to 180°C and bake on the centre shelf for 20–25 minutes or until set and golden. Remove and cool on a wire rack. When the dough has cooled, cut it into pieces or break it apart for a random jagged effect. They are not super crisp, and are quite tender. For a crisper cracker, bake in a 180°C oven for 5–7 minutes just before serving.

5. The biscuits will keep in an airtight container for up to 2 days, so eat them up quickly!

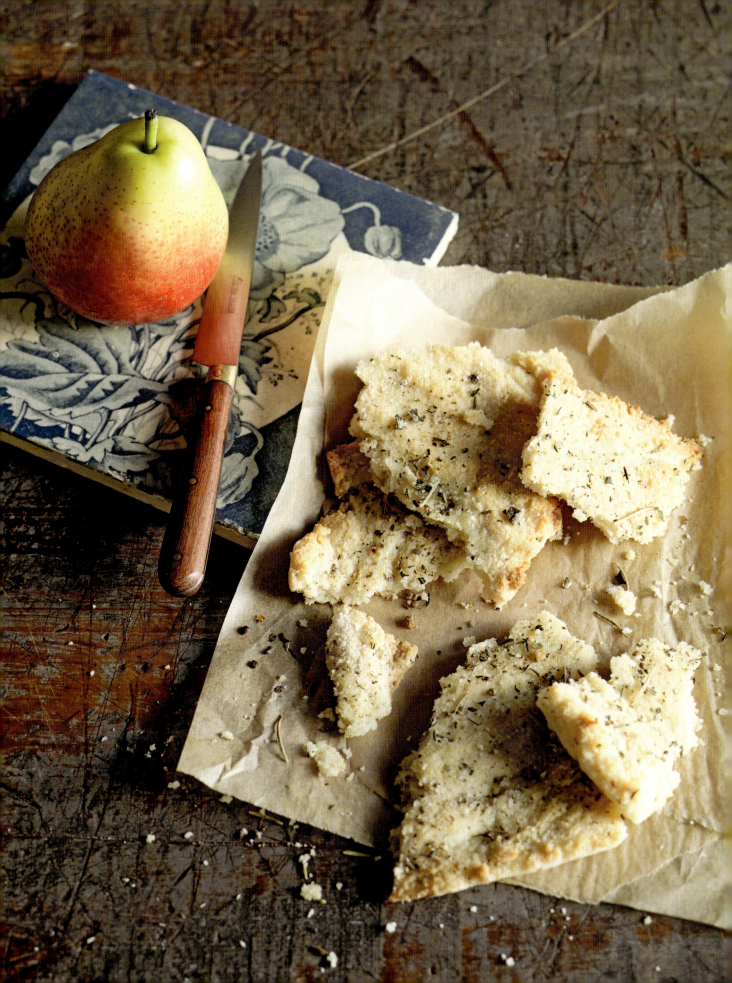

This recipe is the result of pure experimentation driven by a desire to make a soft, flour-free biscuit. I owe its success to my mum – she's the one who worked it out in the end.

Pear and coconut slice

Makes about 15 **PREP TIME:** *15 minutes* **COOKING TIME:** *40 minutes*

---

3 pears
3 eggs
4 cups (320 g) desiccated coconut
3 tablespoons coconut sugar
1 teaspoon vanilla bean powder
pinch of natural salt

1. Preheat the oven at 200°C (fan-forced). Line a baking tray with baking paper.

2. Peel and roughly chop the pears and place in a medium saucepan with 1 cup (250 ml) water. Cover and bring to a simmer over medium heat, then remove from the heat and leave to steam and poach for 5 minutes. Drain, reserving the pear water to make jelly, if liked (see page 202). Set the pears aside to cool, then transfer them to a food processor and puree until smooth.

3. Add the eggs to the pear puree and blend until creamy. Add the desiccated coconut, coconut sugar, vanilla and salt and blend until combined.

4. Spread the mixture on the prepared tray to an even 1 cm thickness. Alternatively, drop 2 tablespoons of mixture per biscuit onto the tray.

5. Reduce the oven temperature to 180°C and bake for 40 minutes. Remove and allow to cool on the tray for 5 minutes, then cut into diagonal biscuits (or use a cookie cutter for different shapes) and transfer to a wire rack to cool completely. Store in an airtight container in the fridge for up to 4 days.

VARIATIONS
Try apples, berries or cherries instead of pears to make a delicious alternative.

To make a chocolate and pear biscuit, add ⅔ cup (70 g) raw cocoa powder to the mixture. These taste like old-fashioned lamingtons!

Fragrant poached fruit

Choose from:

pears, cut into quarters and cored
apples, cut into quarters and cored
rhubarb, chopped
quince, cored and sliced
stone fruit, cut in half and stones removed
berries, whole

1. For every cup of fruit add ½ cup (125 ml) water, 2 teaspoons Fragrant Fruit Spice Blend (or ground cinnamon, nutmeg, clove and hibiscus flower, to taste) and ½ teaspoon vanilla bean powder. For extra sweetness, you might want to add 1 teaspoon coconut sugar, but this depends on the natural sweetness of the fruit.

2. Combine the fruit, water and aromatics in a saucepan and simmer until the fruit is just tender. Cool and keep refrigerated for up to 4 days. Serve with yoghurt or activated nuts and seeds (see pages 218 and 212).

Coconut cream

Open up a young coconut and drain the coconut water into a jar (drink as is or set aside for a smoothie). Scoop out the coconut flesh and puree in a food processor. Store in an airtight container in the fridge for up to 2 days. The coconut cream is delicious as it is, but it may also be flavoured with vanilla bean powder or raw cocoa powder and a pinch of stevia green leaf powder. For a fruity coconut cream, add berries or tropical papaya, banana or pineapple and a squeeze of lime juice.

To make a quick ice-cream, simply spoon coconut cream into a container and freeze. For an even better outcome, use an ice-cream maker.

Homemade 'chocolate'

The traditional art of chocolate making is one that I revere and I have to admit that my homemade version does not replace perfectly roasted chocolate beans that are then ground, conched and tempered to create the highest-quality chocolate. But it does satisfy! The quantities are not specific as it really depends how much you want to make.

Place equal quantities of raw cocoa powder, cocoa butter and coconut oil in a small saucepan. Add a pinch each of stevia green leaf powder and vanilla bean powder and stir gently over low heat until melted and combined. Pour into stainless steel ice-cube trays or chocolate moulds and refrigerate.

Alternatively, dip fruit such as orange segments, strawberries or green apple wedges into the still-warm chocolate and place in the fridge to set.

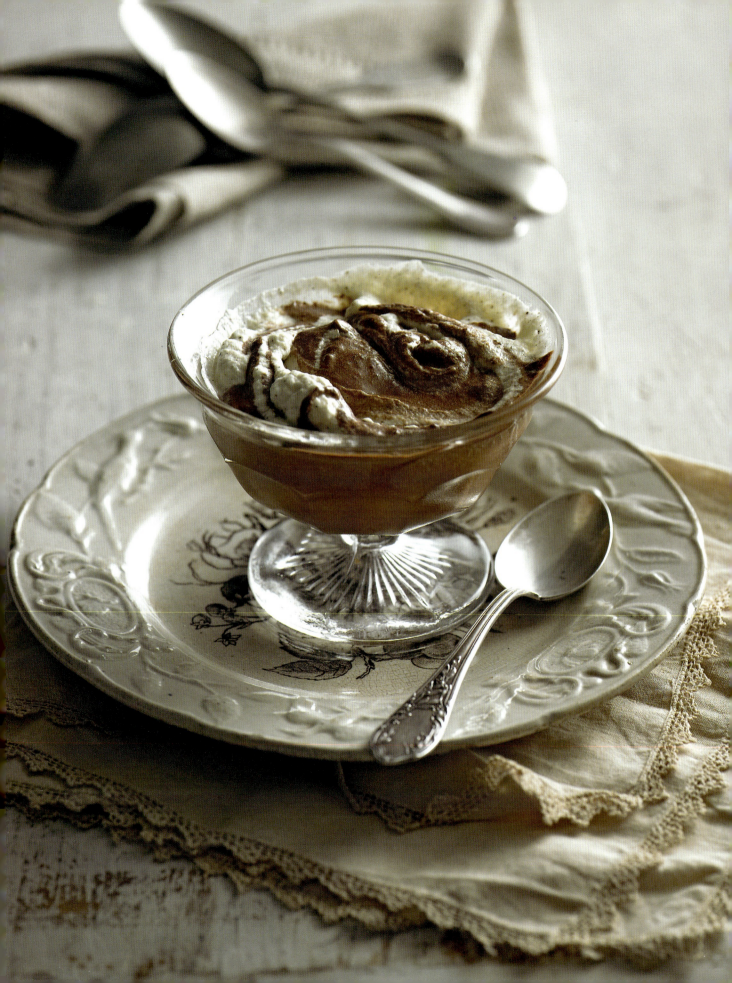

This is so luscious but the only sugar here is found in the chocolate. No other sweeteners are added, so you can enjoy it guilt-free. For a more intense flavour, dust with raw cocoa powder just before serving.

Chocolate mousse

Serves 6 **PREP TIME:** *10 minutes*

---

350 g good-quality dark chocolate, broken into pieces
½ teaspoon vanilla bean powder
4 eggs, separated
200 ml pouring cream, whipped, plus extra to serve

1. Quarter fill a saucepan with water and heat until simmering. Place the chocolate in a heatproof bowl, then set the bowl over the simmering water, but do not allow the base of the bowl to touch the water. Stir until the chocolate has melted, then stir in the vanilla and set aside to cool slightly.

2. In a bowl beat the egg whites until stiff peaks form.

3. Place the egg yolks in another bowl and gently whisk, then add the melted chocolate. Gently fold in the egg whites and whipped cream. Pour into small glasses or cups and enjoy immediately, or refrigerate until ready to serve. Finish with an extra dollop of whipped cream.

VARIATION
To make a quick chocolate ice-cream, scoop the mousse into a container with a lid and freeze. You could also do this in an ice-cream maker, which will give a smoother result.

Real jelly

All recipes serve 2

I used to love eating red jelly at my grandma's house. This was her attempt to give me an Australian treat. It was certainly easy to make; an eager ritual. Open the tiny box of red sugar crystals, pour into a bowl with freshly boiled water, stir until dissolved, pour into pretty glass dishes, put in the fridge and wait anxiously for the red water to set to a fun wobble.

My version is traditional, made from healthy gelatin sources and fresh fruit, juice or fragrant herbal teas. They are free of sugar and artificial additives. I think my darling grandma would approve.

Real gelatin can be obtained by gently boiling grass-fed bones (see Bone stocks on page 214) or you can buy Great Lakes or Bernard Jensen beef gelatin powder. It's natural and grass-fed, derived from the selective hydrolysis of collagen from bovine skin, connective tissue and/or bones. Real gelatin is a healing food for the musculoskeletal system, particularly joints. Jelly is also very cooling, hydrating and soothing for sore throats and fever, heartburn and inflamed digestive conditions. A delicious therapy.

Recipes page 204 >

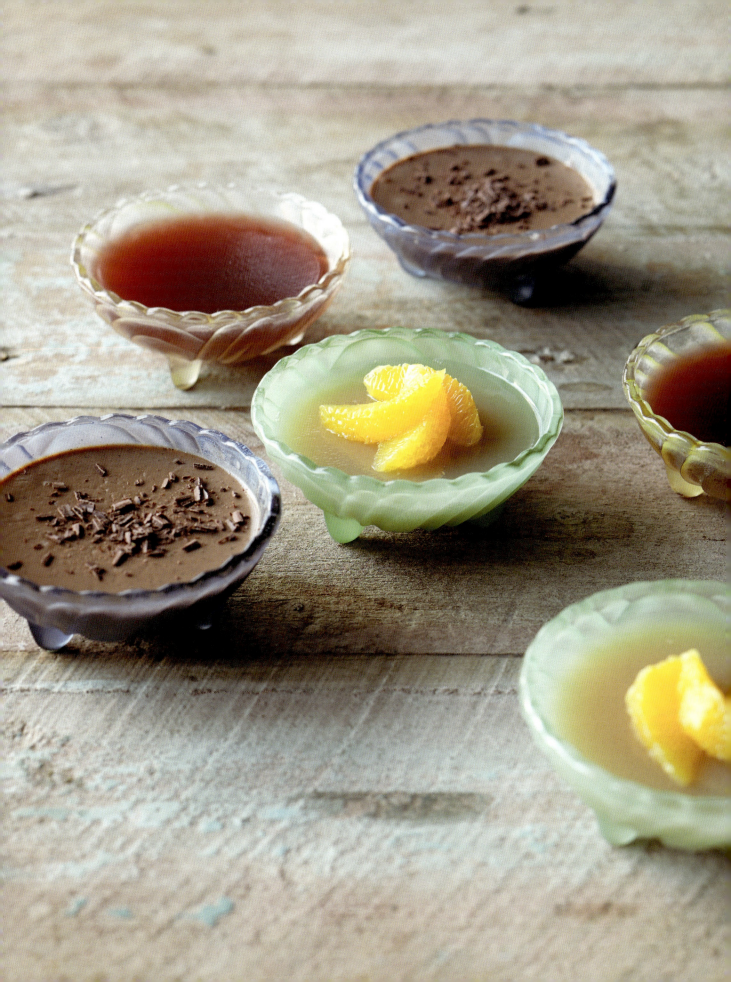

Tea jelly

By choosing a naturally sweet tea blend, there's no need to use sugar. Choose from Vanilla Lemon Heaven Tea, Minty Tea, Summer Pineapple Tea, Vanilla Minty Sky Tea, Paddington Tea or Rise & Shine Tea. Fragrant Fruit Spice Blend with honey also creates a delicate aromatic jelly. Otherwise, choose loose herbs such as licorice root, mint and lemon myrtle.

3 teaspoons herbal tea
400 ml boiling water
1 tablespoon real gelatin powder

1. Spoon the herbal tea into a teapot, add 300 ml boiling water and leave to infuse for 5–7 minutes. Strain into a heatproof jug – this makes it easier to pour the liquid into smaller vessels, such as tea cups or bowls. Combine the gelatin and remaining boiling water and whisk until dissolved, then stir into the tea. Pour into one large bowl or two smaller bowls or cups, then put in the fridge to set.

Fruit jelly

Use whatever freshly made juice you like for this – such as pineapple, pear, apple or berry.

1 tablespoon real gelatin powder
100 ml boiling water
300 ml freshly made fruit juice
about ½ cup diced or sliced fruit (optional)

1. Combine the gelatin and boiling water and whisk until dissolved, then stir into the juice. Add the fresh fruit now, if using, then pour into two small vessels and put in the fridge to set.

Panna cotta

With the simple addition of heat and gelatin you can transform a delicious breakfast smoothie into a delicate, creamy dessert. This is my version of a panna cotta! My favourite is chocolate and coconut milk but any combination from the ingredients on page 81 will turn out beautifully – try banana and almond milk, berry and vanilla or cinnamon and honey.

1 tablespoon real gelatin powder
100 ml boiling water
300 ml freshly made smoothie (see page 81)

1. Combine the gelatin and boiling water and whisk until dissolved, then stir into the smoothie. Pour into two small vessels, then put in the fridge to set.

Jelly made from agar-agar

Agar-agar is a vegetarian 'gelatine' made from a type of algae. Jelly made from agar-agar is stiffer and more solid than jelly made with animal gelatine. Just like gelatine powder, agar-agar doesn't have a flavour and so can easily be used with your choice of flavoured liquid.

2 teaspoons agar-agar powder
100 ml boiling water
300 ml freshly made juice or herbal tea

1. Combine the agar-agar and boiling water and whisk until dissolved, then stir into the juice or tea. Pour into two small vessels and put in the fridge to set.

Kids and adults alike will rejoice in these chewy, yummy, gummy treats and you can dream up any number of familiar or unique flavours to add.

Old-fashioned gummy jellies

Serves 1–4, depending on whether you feel like sharing! **PREP TIME:** *10 minutes, plus setting time*

⅓ **cup (80 ml) flavoursome and naturally colourful liquid, such as tea, juice or smoothie (see page 81)**
3 tablespoons real gelatin powder
3 tablespoons raw honey (if your liquid of choice is not sweet)

1. Pour the liquid into a small saucepan and bring to a simmer, then add the gelatin and stir until dissolved. Taste and sweeten with honey, if needed. Pour into stainless steel moulds made for cookies or hard candy – the smaller the better – and put in the fridge to set. If you don't have small moulds, pour the liquid into a dish or tin to a thickness of 1 cm then simply cut into squares or use a cookie cutter after the jelly has set. Store in the fridge for up to 2 weeks.

VARIATIONS

Sweet and sour gummy jellies
Use freshly squeezed lemon and lime juice and sweeten to taste with honey.

Make a strong pot of Ruby Heart Berry Tea or hibiscus flower tea and sweeten with honey. This has the most fabulous jewel colour.

Sweet gummy jellies
Make a strong pot of tea naturally sweetened with licorice root, such as Vanilla Lemon Heaven or Minty Tea.

Freshly squeezed fruit, such as pear or red apple juice, also makes beautifully sweet gummy jellies. Honey is not needed.

DESSERTS

One of the simplest desserts I know is to imbue succulent seasonal fruit with aromatics such as cinnamon, cardamom, nutmeg, clove, allspice, black pepper, rose, vanilla or green leaf stevia, then serve with yoghurt or cream. This recipe uses one of my favourite ingredients: rosewater, an alluring edible perfume. Unsprayed rose petals make a pretty garnish but they are by no means essential.

Orange, rosewater and pistachio with vanilla yoghurt

Serves 4 **PREP TIME:** *15 minutes, plus chilling time*

3 oranges
3 tablespoons activated pistachios
3 tablespoons rosewater
2 tablespoons raw honey

Vanilla yoghurt

¼ teaspoon vanilla bean powder
1 cup (280 g) homemade (see page 218) or quality store-bought yoghurt

1. Slice the top and bottom off each orange to create a flat surface. Stand the oranges on a chopping board and run the blade of a sharp knife down the inside of the skin, following the shape of the orange and cutting slightly into the flesh. Remove all of the skin and pith, strip by strip, in this way. Place an orange on its side and thinly slice. Arrange the slices on a serving platter and repeat with the remaining oranges.

2. Coarsely chop the pistachios and sprinkle over the oranges. Pour over the rosewater and drizzle with the honey. Set aside in the fridge for 15 minutes to allow the flavours to intermingle and intensify.

3. To make the vanilla yoghurt, combine the vanilla and yoghurt in a small bowl. Serve with the oranges.

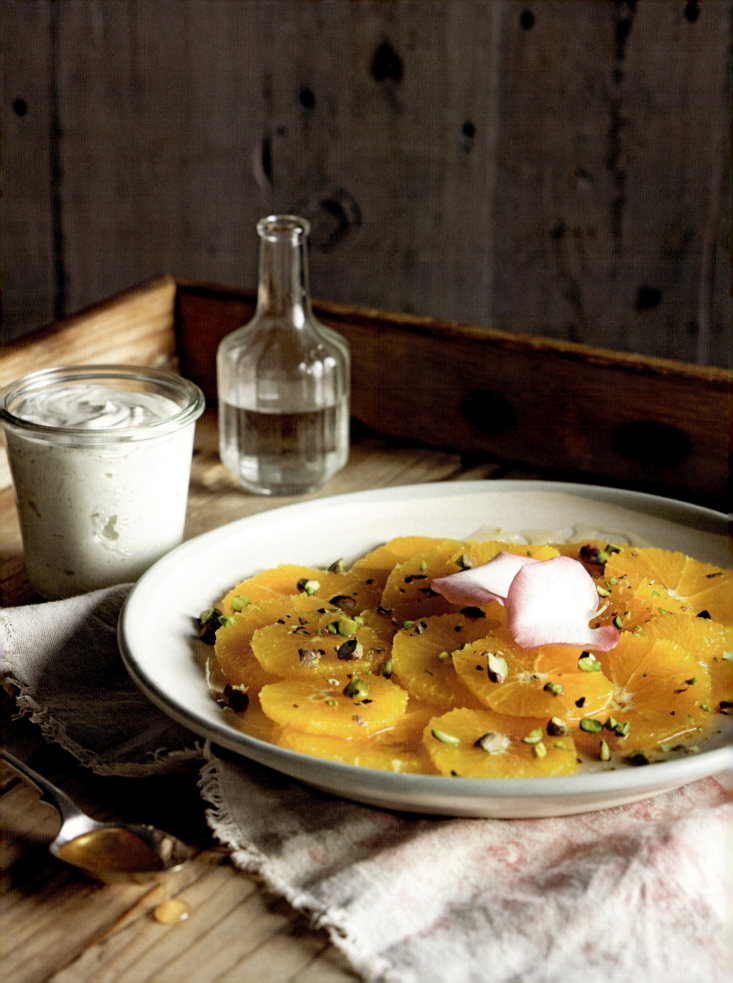

Popsicles are the perfect antidote to heat, and can be made with any seasonal fruit, herbs and spices you like. Gubinge powder, derived from an indigenous Australian plum and available from any health-food store, is the highest natural source of vitamin C on the planet. It is delicious combined with elderflower tea and kiwi, making this popsicle a flavoursome and most enjoyable remedy for a fever.

Elderflower and kiwi popsicles

Makes 6 **PREP TIME:** *15 minutes, plus standing and freezing time*

1 tablespoon elderflower tea
3 tablespoons raw honey
1 tablespoon wildcrafted gubinge powder
3 kiwi fruit, pureed

1. To make the elderflower tea, combine the tea with the honey, gubinge powder and 350 ml boiling water. Stir until the honey has dissolved, then leave to infuse for 10 minutes or until cool. Strain and stir into the pureed kiwi fruit.

2. Pour the mixture into 6 popsicle moulds (preferably stainless steel), leaving a little room at the top for the mixture to expand. Insert the sticks and freeze overnight.

VARIATIONS:

For a creamy popsicle, add some fresh cream or yoghurt (see page 218) or simply use your favourite smoothie recipe (see page 81). Obviously, you can use any fruit you like for these – just make sure they are in season and at their fragrant best. Try:

Watermelon and fresh mint

Pear and ginger

Nectarine and cinnamon

Banana and vanilla

Poached quince and cardamom

You could also add flaked almonds, seeds or chopped fruit for added texture.

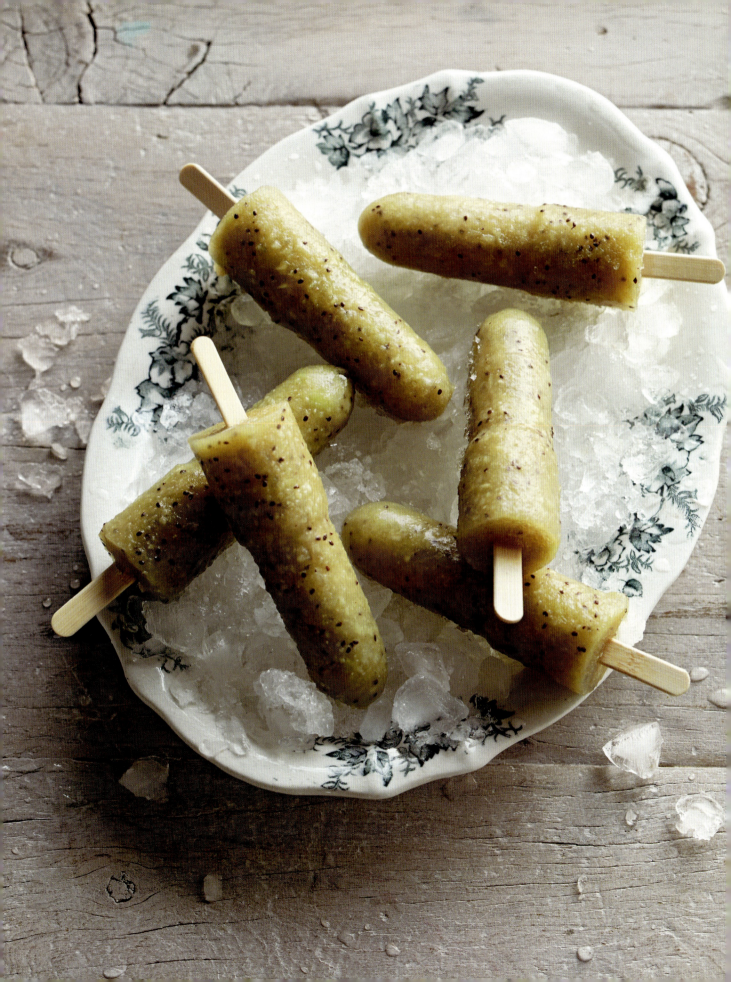

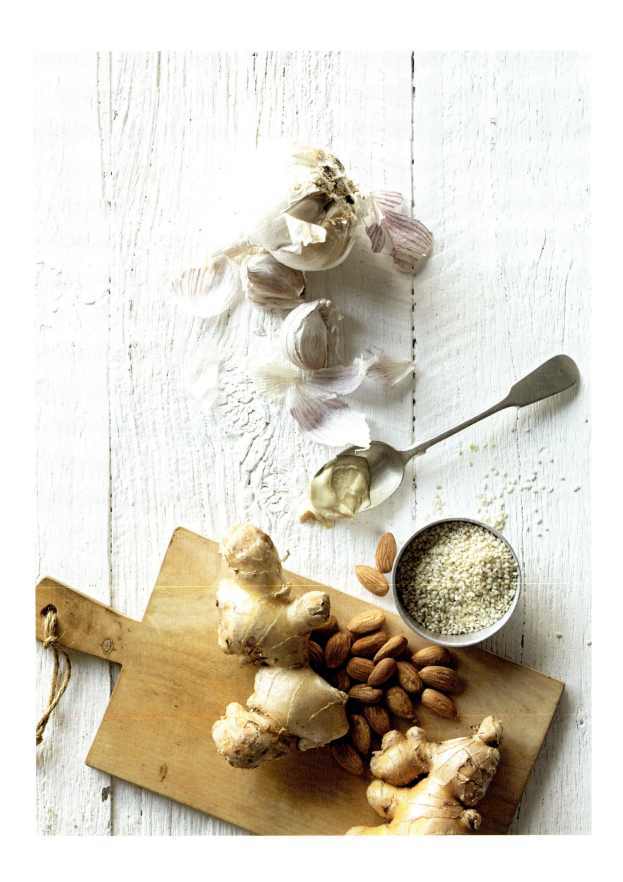

Basics

The recipes in this chapter are homemade goodies that can be made on the weekend or when you have extra time up your sleeve. They range from moreish roasted nuts, stocks and curds to condiments, sauces and pate.

    These basics form the foundation for nutritious meals during the week, speeding up preparation and cooking times after a busy day. In addition, they offer extra nutrition and enhance the digestibility of a meal. Get in the habit of making them regularly for a well-stocked fridge and larder.

Preparing grains, beans, nuts and seeds

In a nutshell (pardon the pun), all grains, beans, nuts and seeds need to be prepared well for nutrient digestion, absorption and assimilation. Refer to pages 34–35 for more information on antinutrients. Preparation is best done over 2 days.

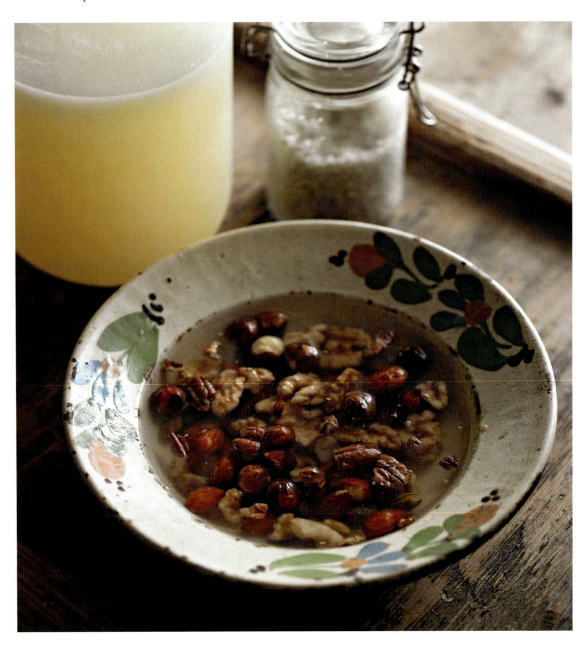

Soaking

Whether you have purchased a wholegrain, rolled flake or flour, soaking in an acid medium is crucial for the elimination of antinutrients, such as phytic acid. An acid medium could be lemon juice, apple cider vinegar or whey (see page 216).

Soak 1 cup of dried material in 3 cups (750 ml) of water with 3–4 tablespoons of acid medium and a pinch of natural salt for at least 12 hours. For nuts and seeds, rinse the next day and dry, then eat as they are or sprout or dry-roast. Brown rice and legumes require extra soaking time.

If you are not going to roast your soaked nuts and seeds immediately, only soak what you are going to eat the next day as they do not store well in or out of the fridge and quickly become mouldy.

NOTE: Almond meal is used in many cake recipes. I specifically choose blanched almond meal to avoid the extra preparation time of soaking. The skin of the almond meal contains the phytic acids.

Roasting

Spread out the soaked nuts and seeds on a baking tray and dry-roast them in a very low oven (40–70°C). This may take all day, but it will give the nuts stability and shelf life. Make sure they are dry and crunchy otherwise they will become mouldy after a couple of days. If you roast at a higher temperature you will destroy the delicate good fats and oils.

Sprouting

Sprouts are a powerhouse of nutrients and are more easily digested than a raw nut, seed, grain or bean. My favourite seeds to sprout are fenugreek, radish, mung, lentil and sunflower. They can be added to a salad or sauteed vegetables.

To grow sprouts in a jar, place 1–2 tablespoons of seeds in a wide-mouth jar, and cover with approximately 5 cm of warm water. Cover the mouth of the jar with muslin or cheesecloth and seal with a rubber band. Let this sit overnight on a kitchen bench. The next day, drain the water and rinse the seeds by adding water to the jar, swishing it around and draining. Repeat twice a day, every day until you have small green sprouts – this may take anywhere from 3 to 7 days. Store your sprouts in a covered bowl with a piece of paper towel inside to absorb excess moisture. Use the sprouts within a week.

Cooking

After soaking legumes and grains in an acid medium for the specified time, rinse them and place in a clean saucepan. Cover with fresh water and simmer until soft. The cooking time will vary but is usually around 30–40 minutes.

Bone stocks

Homemade bone stock is the healthy alternative to processed tetra-packed or canned stock, stock cubes, pastes, liquids or powder. Bone stocks are an essential nutritional food as well as an essential cooking ingredient, making a great base for soups, sauces and roasts.

There are many types of bone stocks: lamb, ham hock, seafood, poultry carcases or whole chicken, beef or marrow. They are all good, and you should allow at least 4–6 hours to do the job properly, or 12 hours in a slow cooker.

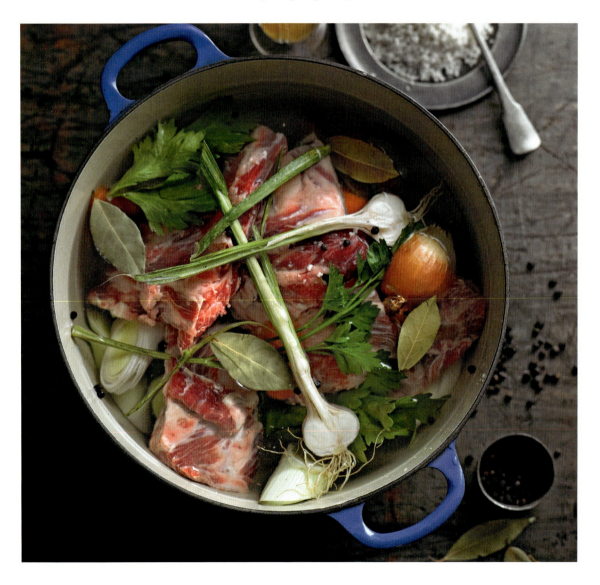

You will need the following ingredients:

Your choice of raw bones or seafood

Water
4 litres for every 1 kg of bones
3.5 litres for every 1.5 kg of whole chicken
3 litres for every 500 g of prawn shells, fish heads and tails

Natural salt
¼ teaspoon for every 1 litre of water

Vegetables
For every 1 kg of bones, add 100 g each of sliced carrot, onion and leek, 1 celery stalk and 1 bunch of flat-leaf parsley stalks

Apple cider vinegar
3 tablespoons for every 1 litre (this will help extract minerals)

1. Place all the ingredients in a large stockpot and simmer, covered, for 4–6 hours (hard or large bones, such as beef bones, can be simmered for up to 10 hours). Skim the froth off the surface every now and then. When the stock is ready, any meat and cartilage will fall off bone. Strain and serve as a clear broth (see page 124) or freeze in 2 cup (500 ml) containers and use as needed.

Bone stocks from leftover bones and bits

Place the congealed fat, gelatin, bones and skin, gravy juices, leftover vegetables and meat in a saucepan. Add extra salt if needed and enough water to cover and simmer, covered, for 2 hours. Skim off any froth that forms on the surface. Drain, discarding the solids. This flavoursome stock can be served as a clear broth or used as a base for stews, casseroles or pilafs.

Gelatin

Gelatin strengthens nails, bones and hair and is excellent for arthritic inflammation. It offers some, but not all, amino acids.

A good-quality bone broth will have plenty of gelatin, which sets like jelly when the bone stock is cold. Beef and marrow bones impart the best gelatin.

To boost the nutrition in your diet, add a few tablespoons of homemade, cold, clear set gelatin made from beef bones to a smoothie (see page 81). If you are doing this, use unflavoured beef or marrow bone stock made from just bones, salt, vinegar and water, or your smoothie will taste most unusual! Alternatively, use a good brand of bovine grass-fed gelatin like Great Lakes (see pages 202–204).

Fresh curds and whey

I don't believe there is a nicer tasting curd than the one you make yourself. A wonderful by-product is the whey, which I use for soaking nuts, seeds, grains and beans and pickling vegetables (see pages 212 and 22). Bring out your inner Miss Muffet with this very easy method for making curds and whey.

Begin with the highest quality unprocessed, organic, full-fat milk, such as raw goat milk or an unhomogenised cow milk. Pour 1 litre of milk into a large glass jar with a wide mouth and cover loosely with a lid to allow carbon dioxide produced in the fermentation process to escape from the jar. Allow it to stand at room temperature for 1–4 days. The weather and temperature of your kitchen will determine how quickly your curds will separate from the whey. If it is very cold, place the jar in a sink filled with warm water for 2 days or so.

Line a large bowl with a clean 100% cotton tea towel (I like to use organic cotton cheesecloth). Pour in the separated milk, then tie up the cloth with tough string and hang on a kitchen cupboard handle with the bowl immediately underneath. The whey will run into the bowl and the curds will collect in the tea towel. Stand for at least several hours. When the whey stops dripping your curd cheese is ready. If liked, you can speed up the process by gently squeezing the curds to release the whey.

Pour the whey into a glass jar with a lid and store in the fridge for up to 6 months. Open up the towel and scrape the curds into a glass container with a lid. Refrigerate and consume within a week.

Savoury curds
Sprinkle flaked natural salt, freshly cracked pepper, a drizzle of olive oil and a ground herb and spice blend of your choice over the curds – I often use the Provincial Herb & Spice Blend, or you can use a mixture of dried rosemary, thyme and sage, to taste. You can even roll the curds into balls and drop them into a jar of olive oil and store in the fridge for up to a week. Spread on celery sticks or crumble into a salad.

Sweet curds
Deliciously aromatic and creamy, these are best made with cow's milk. Add a good pinch of cinnamon powder, vanilla bean powder and stevia green leaf powder to fresh curds. You could also use a little All Things Nice Spice Blend, or a mixture of ground cinnamon, cloves and nutmeg, to taste. Roll into balls if liked and enjoy with berries or green apple slices.

TIP: To replace homemade curds in recipes, use good-quality store-bought full-fat Quark, cream cheese or ricotta.

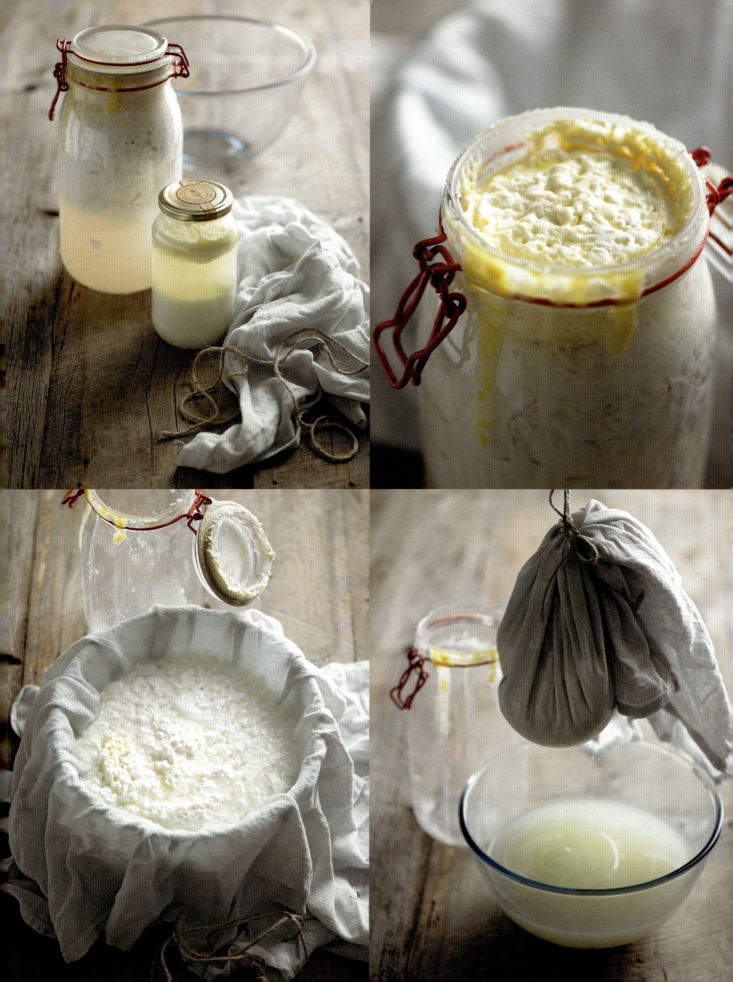

I grew up adding yoghurt to everything I ate. It's something that was always served on our family table alongside salt and pepper – a revered condiment. Making it at home is so incredibly easy that it may soon become a nourishing tabletop garnish in your own household! Even if you choose to buy it, there are excellent store-bought options to rival homemade (albeit less creatively satisfying). Look for yoghurts made with well-sourced milks (from healthy, pastured cows, goats or sheep) prepared using the old-fashioned method of simply combining milk and cultures. Avoid those made from skim milk, milk solids, sugar and other thickeners. (For more information see pages 22, 30 and 40.)

Homemade Greek yoghurt

Makes 1 litre **PREP TIME:** *5 minutes, plus setting time* **COOKING TIME:** *5 minutes*

1 litre full-fat sheep, goat or cow milk, plus 2 tablespoons extra

2 tablespoons homemade yoghurt or plain unflavoured yoghurt with active live cultures

1. Before you start, make sure the milk and yoghurt are both at room temperature.

2. Heat the milk just to boiling point, then pour it into a non-metal container, sitting on a towel. Let it cool until lukewarm; a skin will form on top. Mix the yoghurt with the extra milk, then add it to the lukewarm milk, carefully pouring it down the side so that any skin that may have formed is not disturbed. Gently swirl the container around to mix the yoghurt into the milk, taking care not to disturb the skin. Cover with a clean tea towel and place on another towel in a warm, dry place to thicken for at least 8 hours or overnight (12 hours is best). The longer the yoghurt coagulates beyond that time, the more sour the taste becomes.

3. Carefully drain off any excess liquid (whey), then pour it into a glass jar with a lid and store in the fridge for up to 6 months. Use the whey for culturing vegetables or soaking nuts, seeds, grains and beans (see pages 221 and 212).

4. Spoon the yoghurt into a glass jar with a lid and refrigerate for 4 hours before using. It will keep in the fridge for 4–5 days. Don't forget to save a small amount to make the next batch!

5. If you prefer a thicker yoghurt, strain it in a muslin cloth.

Aphrodite's delight
Drizzle raw honey over a bowl of Greek yoghurt and sprinkle with chopped activated walnuts, pistachios and pomegranate seeds or fresh figs.

For other delicious ways to serve yoghurt, see pages 81 and 82.

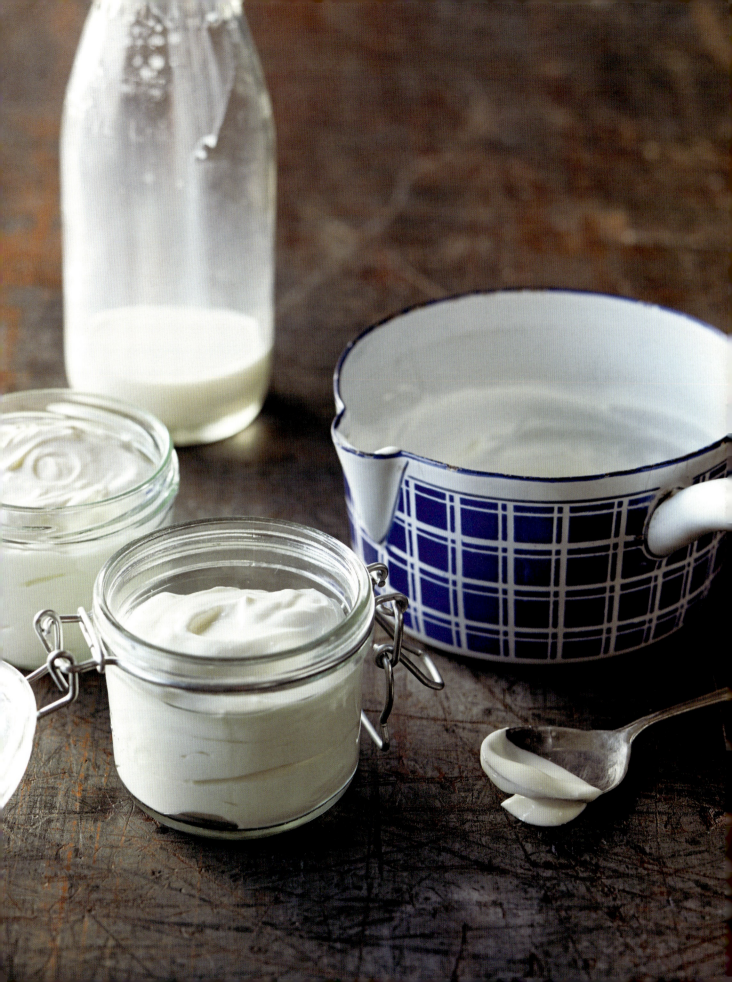

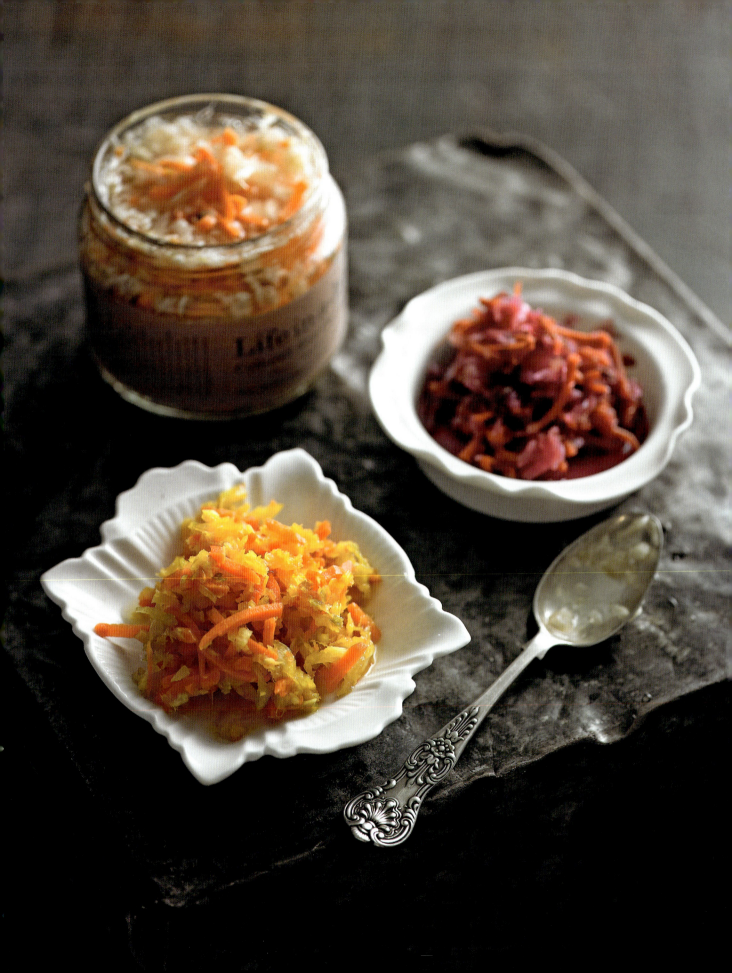

Cultured vegetables

Cultured vegetables were traditionally prepared to preserve food for a longer shelf life, but we now know that they also offer an array of nutritional and health benefits (such as live enzymes to aid digestion and good bacteria). If you are allergic to dairy, add an extra tablespoon of salt in place of the whey. Serve cultured vegetables with meat or eggs, or add to a salad to give it a zing!

Fermented cabbage, carrots and caraway seeds

½ cabbage, shredded
2 carrots, shredded
1 tablespoon natural salt
⅓ cup (80 ml) whey (see page 216 or 218)
1 teaspoon caraway seeds

1. Place all the ingredients in a bowl and mix well. Transfer to a 1 litre wide-mouth jar and pound with a mallet in the jar to release the juices. Add 1 cup (250 ml) water, leaving 2–3 cm at the top of the jar as the vegetables will expand. Secure the lid, then leave the jar in a warm place for 3–6 days to ferment. During this fermentation period, the friendly bacteria will reproduce and convert sugars and starches to lactic acid. The fermentation time very much depends on the weather – it is closer to 3 days in warm conditions, but could take up to 6 days when it is cool. Refrigerate for up to 2 months.

VARIATIONS

Add turmeric powder for a strong anti-inflammatory effect.

Add grated ginger, chilli or garlic for an antimicrobial and anti-inflammatory effect.

Fennel or dill seeds may be used instead of caraway seeds to soothe and aid digestion.

Vary the vegetables to suit your tastes. Other vegetables that pickle well are celery, capsicum (pepper), beetroot, daikon and cucumber.

Pickled ginger

1.4 kg younger ginger root (skin on) or peeled older ginger root, very thinly sliced with a mandolin
1 tablespoon natural salt
⅓ cup (80 ml) whey (see page 216 or 218)

1. Place the ginger in a medium wide-mouth jar and pound with a mallet in the jar to release the juices. Mix together the salt, whey and 1 cup (250 ml) water and pour into the jar, leaving 2–3 cm at the top of the jar as the ginger will expand. Secure the lid, then leave the jar in a warm place for 3 days to ferment. Refrigerate for up to 2 months. Serve with raw fish (see page 136) and salads.

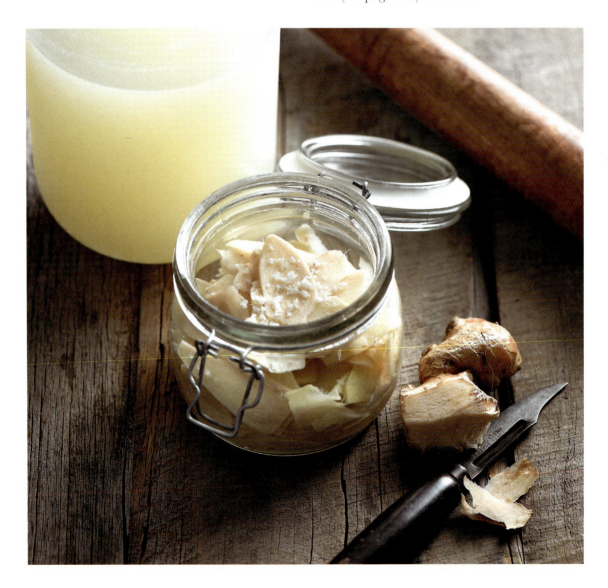

Kefir yoghurt drink

This delicious sour drink, made with kefir grain culture, is an excellent source of good bacteria. Traditionally, kefir grains are obtained from an existing kefir yoghurt drink where they naturally multiply and grow. Look online for a source of real kefir grain culture, which will be sent in a little ready-made kefir. Alternatively, ask a friend who has a batch to share some with you.

Add 1 tablespoon of kefir grains to 2 cups (500 ml) organic, whole unprocessed milk or other liquid mediums such as coconut water, and leave to ferment with lid on loosely. Store the culture out of direct sunlight in the warmest spot in your kitchen for 24 hours, then strain it through a sieve using a fork to separate the kefir yoghurt from the grains. Pour the yoghurt back in the jar, then store in the fridge and consume within a week. Add your new batch of kefir grain culture to fresh milk and begin the process again. Kefir grain cultures needs a medium as they will die as soon as they dry out. Drink kefir yoghurt as is, add it to smoothies or make a deliciously tart salad dressing by combining equal parts of olive oil and kefir yoghurt, then seasoning with natural salt and freshly cracked pepper.

Beet kvass

This is another traditional lactofermented drink full of live enzymes and healthy bacteria that can aid digestion and cleanse the liver. This delicious, refreshing drink can also be used as a salad dressing instead of vinegar – simply whisk it with olive oil and freshly cracked pepper.

3 beetroots, peeled and roughly chopped
1 tablespoon natural salt
½ cup (125 ml) whey (see page 216 or 218)

1. Place all the ingredients in a 1 litre jar and add enough water to cover, leaving 2–3 cm at the top of the jar as the beetroot mixture will expand. Secure the lid, then leave the jar in a warm place for 2 days if you have a very warm kitchen, and up to a week in winter or if your kitchen is cold. Refrigerate for up to 2 months. When all the kvass liquid has been consumed, fill up the jar with fresh water and leave to ferment out of the fridge for a further 2 days, or more if it's cold. Refrigerate and consume until complete, then discard the beetroot as a third extraction will not yield any more goodness.

2. For therapeutic purposes drink one glass upon rising and one before dinner.

Nothing beats the flavour of homemade mayonnaise, and the beauty is it's so simple to make, especially if you use a food processor. Choose a Dijon mustard that is made simply from mustard seeds, apple cider vinegar, natural salt and water.

Mayonnaise

Makes about 1⅔ cups (420 ml) **PREP TIME:** *10 minutes*

2 large egg yolks
2 tablespoons apple cider vinegar
1½ tablespoons Dijon mustard
380 ml extra virgin olive oil
1–2 tablespoons fresh lemon juice
½ teaspoon natural salt, or to taste

1. Process the egg yolks, vinegar and mustard in a food processor, then very slowly add the olive oil in a steady stream until the mixture becomes creamy. Add the lemon juice and salt, to taste. Store in the fridge in an airtight container for up to 1 week.

VARIATIONS

For a herb mayonnaise add a good handful of finely chopped fresh herbs, such as tarragon, flat-leaf parsley and thyme.

To make an aioli, add 1 clove of crushed garlic at the same time as the lemon juice.

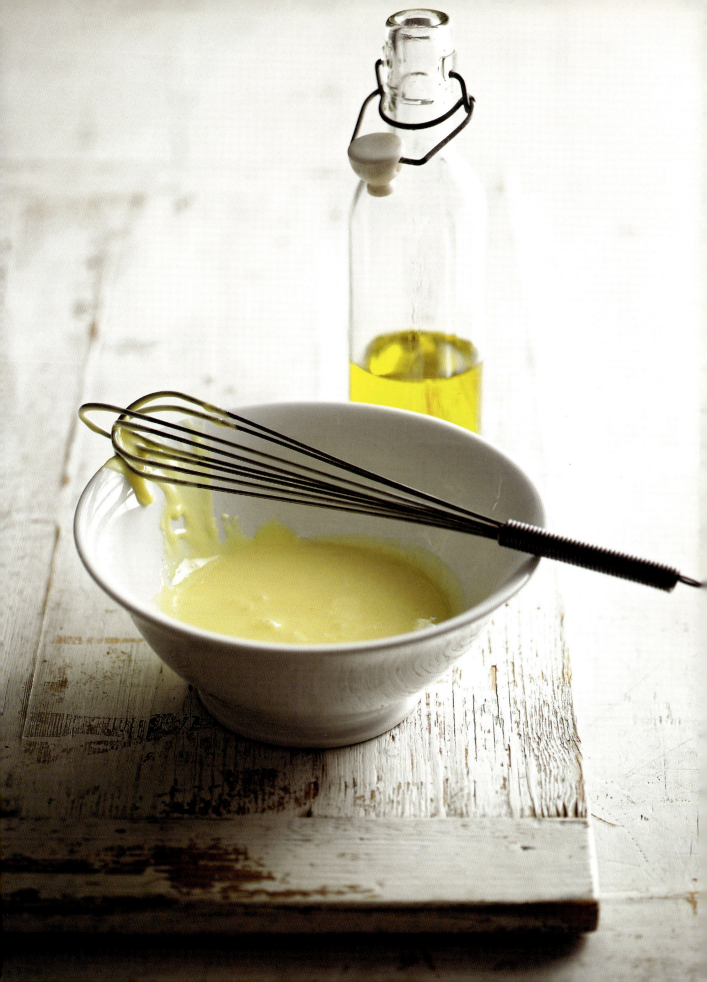

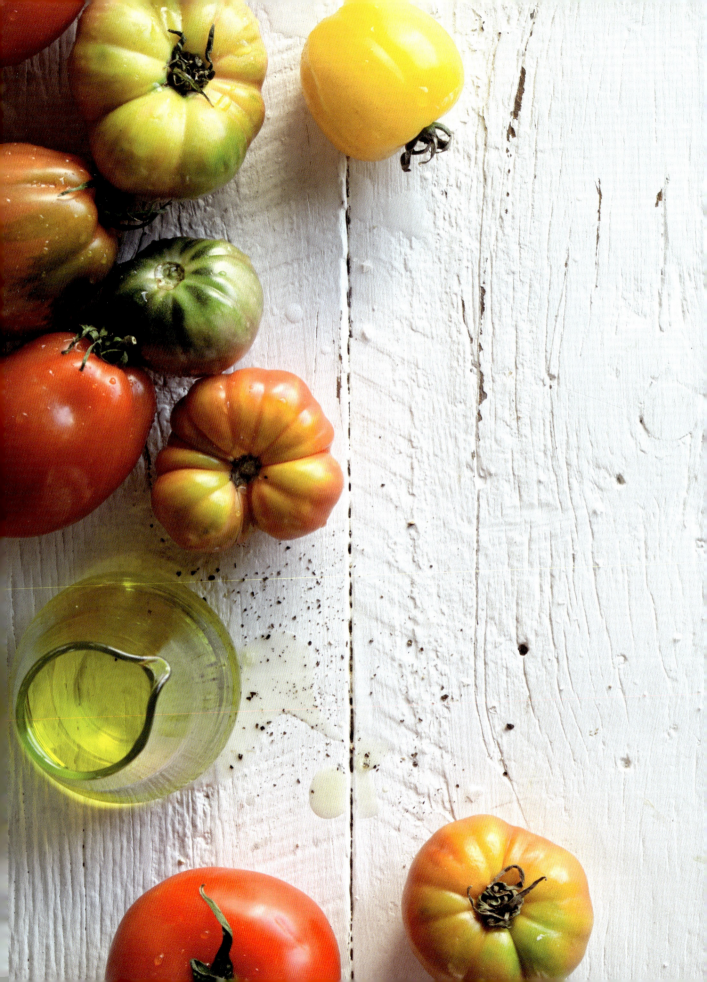

Store-bought tomato sauce is full of sugar and processed additives. I don't want to go without, as I love, love, love serving it with steak and sausages, so I developed my own recipe. I hope you will love it too!

Tomato sauce

Makes 2 litres **PREP TIME:** *20 minutes* **COOKING TIME:** *1 hour 20 minutes*

---

2 kg vine-ripened tomatoes, green part removed, cut in half
3 tablespoons olive oil
Tuscan Herb & Spice Blend or a blend of dried oregano, basil and marjoram, to taste
natural salt and freshly cracked pepper
1 onion, finely chopped
2 cloves garlic, crushed
apple cider vinegar, to taste

1. Preheat the oven to 220°C (fan-forced).

2. Place the tomatoes, cut-side up, in a large roasting tin. Drizzle with 2 tablespoons olive oil, then sprinkle over the spice blend and season with salt and pepper. Reduce the oven temperature to 120°C and roast the tomatoes for 30–50 minutes or until softened and starting to collapse. The actual cooking will depend on the size of the tomatoes.

3. Meanwhile, heat the remaining olive oil in a large saucepan over low heat, add the onion and cook until softened. Add the garlic and stir for 1 minute more. Add the roast tomatoes and juices and cook, stirring occasionally, for 20–30 minutes or until thick and reduced. Add apple cider vinegar, to taste.

4. Puree and bottle while the sauce is still hot, then store in the fridge for up to a week. Adding olive oil to the top of the sauce after every use will further preserve it.

A natural superfood, liver is one of the most nutrient-dense foods available to us. Yes, liver! Rich in protein, water-soluble vitamins B12, B9, iron and fat-soluble vitamins A and D, it offers complete nutrition in a digestible form, far above any supplement or processed super food. Prior to synthetic supplementation, liver was used as a remedy for many nutritional deficiencies such as anaemia or general malnutrition, recovery from an operation, stress and convalescence. This is an instant, pick-me-up food!

Liver gets a bad rap as it is the organ of detoxification. Choose liver from an organic and pastured source and it will be free of chemicals, antibiotics and hormones. With a better understanding of what it takes to raise healthy animals comes respect and gratitude for the whole animal, including its organs. They should never be discarded but added to our diet, just as we use animal bones for stocks and animal fat for cooking.

Pate is the way I like to eat liver – in fact, I highly recommend making a batch every week. The liver may come from a chicken, duck, lamb or calf – it's entirely up to you. My favourite is this chicken liver pate. Eat it with carrot, celery or cucumber sticks, and stir any leftovers into soups and stocks.

Chicken liver pate

Serves 2 as a light meal or 6 as a canape **PREP TIME:** *15 minutes* **COOKING TIME:** *10 minutes*

---

100 g quality cultured butter or ghee
3–4 cloves garlic, crushed
1 red or brown onion or 1 leek, roughly chopped
500 g organic chicken livers, trimmed
2 teaspoons Tuscan Herb & Spice Blend or dried oregano, basil and marjoram, to taste

1. Melt 40 g butter or ghee in a medium frying pan, add the garlic and onion or leek and cook for 5 minutes or until soft and transparent. Add the liver and spice blend and saute for a couple of minutes until just cooked, but not brown all the way through. Their colour will turn from burgundy blood-red to an opaque, brownish pink. A grey-brown colour means that they are over-cooked and will not taste as good.

2. Allow to cool slightly, then process in a food processor until smooth. Add 40 g butter or ghee and process again. Pour into a 700 ml glass jar with a lid and smooth the surface with the back of a spoon. Melt the remaining butter or ghee, then pour evenly over the pate to seal – this helps preserve the pate for longer. Allow to cool completely, then serve or refrigerate for up to 7 days.

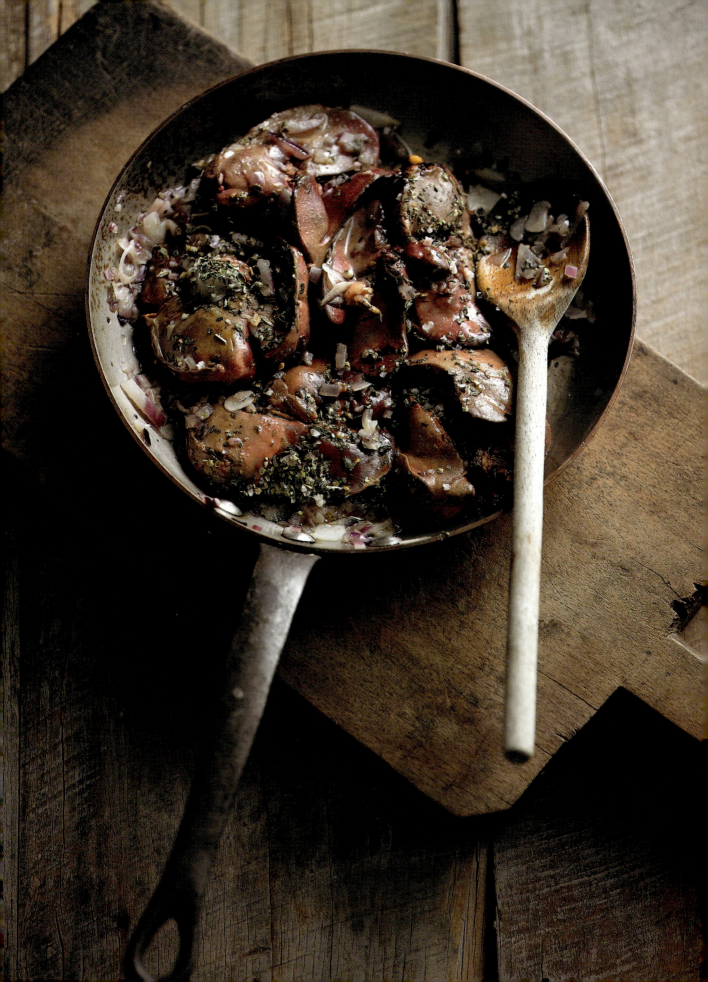

Herbal teas

At the end of a long day I love to enjoy a cup of herbal tea just as is, or with a small bite of something, such as a coconut macaroon (see page 184) that won't raise my blood sugar levels before bed. I created my range of Ovvio organic teas for myself and for clients to enjoy. My favourite bedtime teas are Peace Bambino Tea and Chamomile Nights Tea.

Ovvio organic teas are therapeutically blended according to the principles of traditional herbal medicine. Each tea offers an emotional, physical and mental health benefit of calm, energy, clarity, restoration or detoxification. The following teas are a small sample from my range, some of which may be used in the recipes.

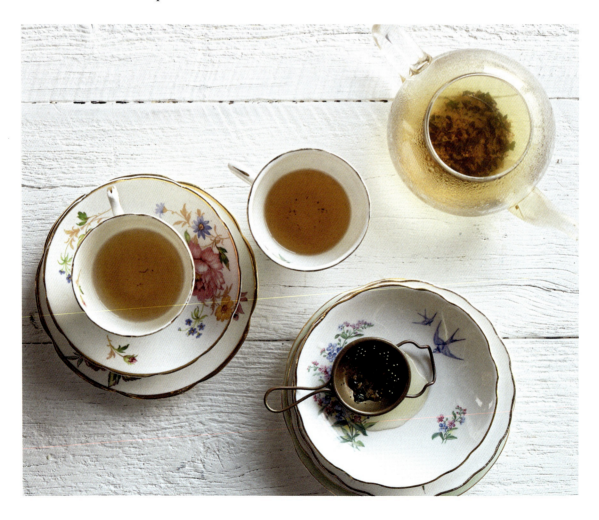

C-Strength Citrus Tea
Vitamin C-rich orange, elderberry, rosehip and licorice for the adrenal glands and immunity.

Chamomile Nights Tea
Give yourself a tranquil night with this blend of hops, passionflower, lavender and chamomile.

Clarity Sage Tea
Sage, mint, rosemary and lavender. Traditionally used for headaches, focus and memory.

D-Tox Bitters Tea
Milk thistle, artichoke leaf, cinnamon and fennel. Traditionally used for a bowel and liver detox, digestion and fat metabolism.

Dandy Chai Tea
Dandelion root with warming, aromatic clove, cinnamon, fennel, ginger and cardamom.

Derma-Kleanze Tea
Purify and clear the skin with rose, lemon myrtle and other blood-purifying herbs.

Happy Bowels Tea
A gentle cleanse for the bowels with licorice, spearmint, dandelion and fennel.

Minty Tea
Mint and licorice to freshen the palate and enliven the senses.

Nourish Aromatic Spice Tea
Aniseed, fennel, clove, ginger and cinnamon to gently warm you up from the inside out.

Paddington Tea
Australian lemon myrtle, lemongrass and licorice. Similar actions to Rise and Shine.

Peace Bambino Tea
Chamomile, aniseed, caraway and dill. Gives solace to a breast-feeding mum and baby.

Pure-ify Tea
An all-round systemic cleanser with green hops, rooibos, dandelion, lemon myrtle and linden.

Rise & Shine Tea
A wake-up blend of lemon myrtle, lemongrass, licorice and ginger zing.

Ruby Heart Berry Tea
Juniper, hibiscus flowers and rosehip to improve circulation and harmonise the heart.

Spring Elderflower Tea
Elder, olive leaf, eyebright, lemon, mint and linden flower for sinus problems and hayfever.

Summer Pineapple Tea
A sweet balmy tea of lemons, pineapple, mint and licorice. Drink warm or as a cool iced tea.

Vanilla Lemon Heaven Tea
Luscious lemony herbs, sweet licorice and smooth vanilla. Satisfies sugar cravings.

Vanilla Mint Sky Tea
A cool fusion of peppermint and smooth vanilla. Dream of Monet's sky.

Winter Olive Tea
Olive, mint, lemon, elder and eyebright. Brighten a wintry day with this nurturing tea.

> **TO MAKE PERFECT TEA**
> Boil water and add to your cup to warm. Place 1 teaspoon of tea for every 1 cup (250 ml) of water in a teapot or infuser.
>
> **Specific infusion times**
> **Delicate and floral (leaves, petals or white tea):** Let the boiled water sit and cool for 30 seconds before pouring. Steep for 1–3 minutes before serving.
>
> **Robust and hearty (twigs, bark, roots, buds, seeds and pods):** Steep for 5–7 minutes to extract the goodness from these more hardy ingredients.
>
> **Black, green and everything in between:** Steep for 2–5 minutes and allow the tea leaves to unfurl and mature.

Seasonings

Salt and pepper
The quintessential staples to season any food are salt (see page 49 for the best salt choices) and pepper. Whether they are added during or after cooking, these two ingredients enhance the flavour of any meal.

Salt
Salt not only enhances the flavour of food, it aids digestion and adds nutrition in the form of minerals.

I have specified natural salt throughout the book, and this includes unrefined sea salt, rock salt, river salt and cave salt.

Pepper
Pepper adds a spicy heat to food due to its piperine compound. There are three types of pepper from the same plant:

black pepper (cooked and dried unripe fruit)

green pepper (dried unripe fruit)

white pepper (dried ripe seeds)

Of the three, black pepper is the most commonly used.

A pink peppercorn is a dried berry of the Peruvian peppertree shrub rather than the black peppercorn vine. They are so named because they resemble peppercorns and have a peppery flavour.

It is preferably to buy whole peppercorns and grind them yourself as needed, as oxidation begins when you grind and expose them to oxygen. Freshly cracked pepper releases a more woody, warm and robust aroma and flavour.

Fresh herbs
Fresh herbs transform simple ingredients into something special, adding a fresh but intense layer of flavour. They are easy to grow in your garden and offer antioxidant and therapeutic benefits.

Dried herbs have a more intense flavour than fresh so generally it's best to use double the quantity of fresh herbs to dried herbs or spices. For example, 2 teaspoons of fresh oregano leaves is equal to 1 teaspoon of dried oregano leaves.

Below are a few combinations that create flavours we are all familiar with, simply, elegantly and free of a bottle or paste.

INGREDIENTS THAT MARRY WELL

Vietnamese basil, coriander root and leaves, lemongrass, garlic, ginger root, galangal root and chilli. These fresh ingredients are delicious in a coconut soup, crisp salad with fish or a fresh herb salad dressing made with coconut oil, lime juice, lime zest, natural salt and pepper.

Turmeric root, bay leaves, curry leaves, ginger root, garlic and chilli. Saute these fresh herbs in ghee, add your choice of diced meat and vegetables and serve with a cooling Minty cucumber yoghurt dip (see page 98).

Flat-leaf parsley, basil, oregano, marjoram and garlic. These work beautifully in tomato-based dishes.

Rosemary, oregano and garlic. This simple combination adds Mediterranean flavours to lamb stews or meatballs.

See also pages 234–39 for information on dried herbs and spices.

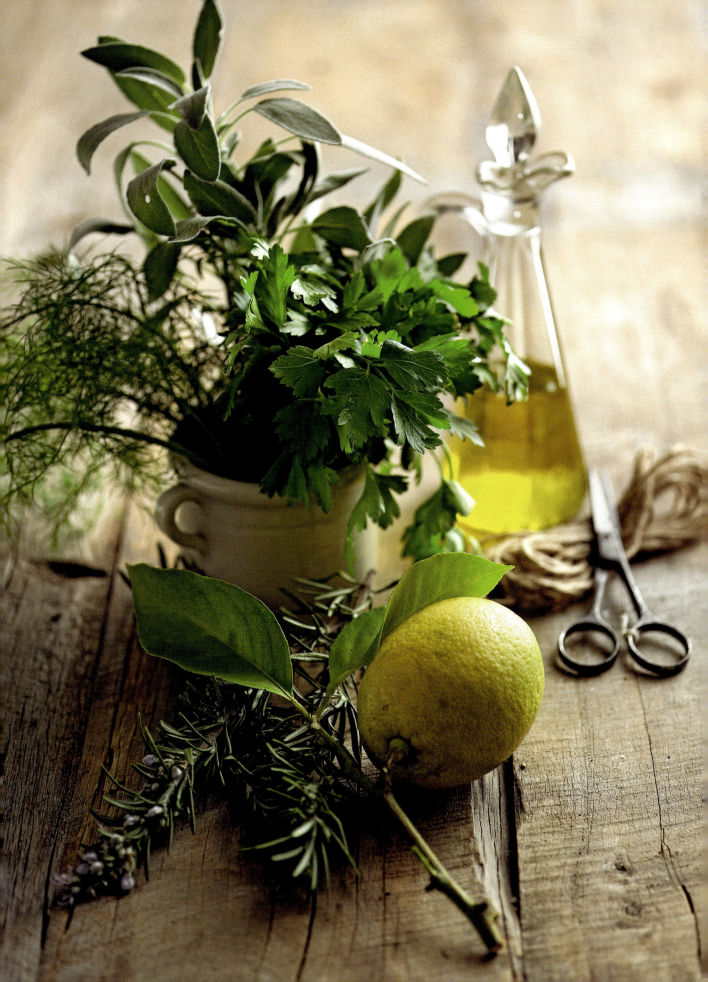

A–Z of dried herbs and spices

I love all herbs and spices – I guess it comes with the territory of being a herbalist. I love them for their ability to transform beautiful ingredients into a delicious and therapeutic meal. Embrace edible medicine and heal thyself, naturally.

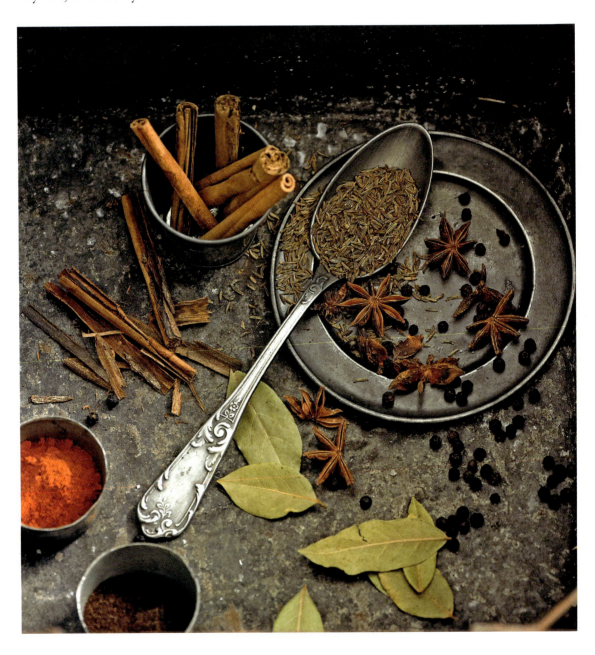

Allspice powder is a warm spice that has the flavour of cinnamon, cloves and nutmeg. Use it in baking, yoghurt or smoothies. Therapeutically augments the digestion by increasing enzyme secretions in the stomach and intestines. It aids flatulence and tummy discomfort and acts as an antiseptic.

Aniseed is similar to fennel seeds, and has a sweet, warm aroma and a slight licorice taste. Use it in sweet or savoury cooking. Therapeutically acts as an expectorant and soothes persistent coughs and a sore tummy. Drink it as a warming tea.

Bay leaves have a sweet, balsamic and spicy scent and flavour for roasts, curries and soups. One or two leaves is all you need in a dish. Therapeutically, bay leaves soothe the tummy.

Basil adds a warm and sweet flavour to tomato dishes. It blends particularly well with oregano and marjoram. Therapeutically the natural essential oils give this herb anti-infective and anti-inflammatory properties.

Caraway seeds have a pungent, anise-like flavour and are used in sweet dishes, savoury roasts or to pickle or lactoferment vegetables. Therapeutically soothes a sore tummy and is indicated for congestive coughs. Drink as a warming tea.

Cardamom pods add a sweet, warm, exotic flavour to curries, puddings and poached fruit. Therapeutically soothes a sore tummy and stimulates circulation. Drink as a warming tea.

Cayenne pepper powder is a ground chilli pepper that adds heat to dishes. Therapeutically acts as an appetite suppressant and metabolism booster.

Chilli flakes add a bite of heat to dishes – sprinkle on food along with salt flakes and cracked pepper just before serving a meal. Therapeutically acts as an appetite suppressant and metabolism booster.

Cinnamon powder, chips and quills bring a sweet, spicy, warm and fragrant note to sweet and savoury dishes. Add to roast pumpkin, poached fruit, yoghurt or smoothies. Therapeutically indicated for colds and flu and digestive upsets.

Clove buds are a rich aromatic that work well with cinnamon, fennel and ginger. They are particularly lovely with roast pork belly and apples. Therapeutically a simple clove bud placed in the mouth will impart analgesic effects for tooth pain. Relieves digestive issues and has antimicrobial effects.

Coriander seeds add a warm, spicy and citrusy note to curries, sauteed meat or vegetables with chilli. Therapeutically soothes the digestion, like many aromatic warming spices.

Cumin seeds encapsulate the taste of India. Use them in curries with fenugreek and turmeric or Mexican blends with chilli and oregano. Therapeutically soothes the digestion, like many aromatic warming spices.

Dill seeds taste like fennel and celery seeds with a hint of citrus. Delicious with fish or pickled vegetables. Therapeutically acts as a digestive tonic and soothes the tummy; especially indicated for infants and babies.

Fennel seeds lend a licorice flavour to sweet or savoury curry dishes or roasted vegetables and garlic. Therapeutically acts as a digestive tonic and soothes the tummy; especially indicated for infants and babies. Encourages milk flow in breast-feeding mothers. Also indicated for upper respiratory issues. Drink as a warming tea.

Fenugreek seeds have a distinctive curry flavour, and are often used with turmeric, ginger, cinnamon and cardamom. Therapeutically warming and indicated to encourage milk flow in breast-feeding mothers as well as regulate blood sugar levels. A nutritive, and indicated for loss of appetite.

Garlic granules offer the pungency and potency of garlic in its dry form. Very convenient when fresh is not available. Therapeutically indicated for infection, colds and flu due to its antimicrobial properties.

Ginger root adds warmth, spice and sweetness. It is often used in Oriental and Indian-style cooking, and is delicious with pork or duck. Therapeutically indicated for nausea and digestive upsets and to warm a cold constitution. Like chilli, it stimulates the metabolism.

Juniper berries have a sweet and spicy pine aroma. Use them when roasting chicken and making other poultry dishes. Therapeutically indicated for digestive upset, cystitis and rheumatism.

Lavender flower add a floral bouquet to any sweet dish. Therapeutically it is antidepressant and antispasmodic, soothing digestive upset, anxiety and headaches. It is indicated for insomnia. Drink as a tea or make a jelly.

Lemon myrtle offers a vibrant lemon flavour and scent that is perfect for fish or chicken. Therapeutically indicated for the common cold, flu, bronchitis, indigestion and other irritable digestive disorders. Drink as a warming tea.

Marjoram smells very Italian and marries well with oregano and basil for any tomato dish. Therapeutically indicated for digestive upset.

Mustard seeds add warmth and heat to a dish. Gently toast black or yellow seeds in a dry pan with some Indian Herb & Spice Blend (or a curry leaf and ground cumin, turmeric and fenugreek, to taste). Add ghee, onions, meat and vegetables for a simple but delicious curry. Therapeutically, its stimulating, diaphoretic action can also be utilised for fevers, colds and flu.

Nutmeg is warm and sweet, perfect in a savoury cheese and spinach pie or warm milk. Combines perfectly with stevia, cinnamon and vanilla.

Oregano is most often found in Italian and Greek cooking. It is the quintessential herb for any tomato dish. Therapeutically similar to thyme but not as intense in its actions.

Paprika powder can be sweet, hot or smoky, offering a mild or hot heat for chicken or fish dishes. Also lovely sprinkled over dips. Shares similar therapeutic properties to cayenne but is much, much milder. It is a source of vitamin C.

Parsley leaf is best used as a fresh garden salad herb or to garnish or complete any Mediterranean dish. Therapeutically it is anti-inflammatory, boosts immunity and has diuretic, cleansing effects.

Peppercorns are readily available in both black and white. Therapeutically acts as a digestive tonic, like many aromatic warming spices.

Peppermint has a sweet, fresh flavour that is delicious in cucumber yoghurt dips or added to a Greek tomato and haloumi salad. Therapeutically cools the constitution and soothes the digestive system.

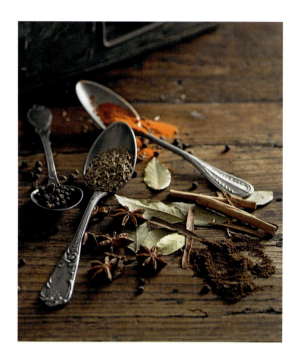

Rosemary has a woody scent that works really well in any lamb dish or liver pate. Therapeutically, it has antimicrobial, analgesic (pain-relieving), antioxidant and antispasmodic properties and stimulates detoxification. It can be made into a tea to increase mental concentration, calm constrictive headaches, anxiety, colic and wind. It is also wonderful for memory – which is why rosemary is worn on Remembrance Day.

Sage leaves have a pine, woody fragrance suitable for stuffings, fish dishes and scrambled eggs with thyme. Therapeutically its antiseptic properties are indicated for gingivitis, sore throats and tonsillitis. Add 2 teaspoons dried sage leaves to 1 cup (250 ml) boiled water to make an excellent mouthwash or gargle. It can also be employed for night sweats.

Star anise adds a pungent aromatic licorice flavour to poached fruit or Oriental dishes such as roast duck or pork. Therapeutically indicated for digestive upset and coughs. The seeds act as an effective breath freshener.

Stevia green leaf powder is a naturally sweet herb that doesn't raise blood sugar levels and has no calorie yield. Only a pinch is needed. It is perfect with vanilla and cinnamon in yoghurt and smoothies.

Thyme has a leafy, lemony flavour. Use it with sage for Mediterranean recipes. Therapeutically significant as an antiseptic, antimicrobial and antispasmodic, indicated for ailments of the digestive and respiratory system.

Turmeric powder gives curry powder its distinctive flavour. It is so medicinal that it is used to prevent and treat many inflammatory conditions. Therapeutically it is anti-inflammatory, antioxidant and liver protective. It is indicated for many chronic illnesses.

Vanilla bean powder gives a smooth, luscious quality to foods, evoking old-fashioned milkshakes and grandma's homemade desserts. Use it in smoothies, yoghurt, poached fruit and baking to lend a naturally sweet, heavenly smooth flavour. Therapeutically and historically employed as an aphrodisiac.

Dried herb and spice blends

This is my collection of Ovvio Organic herb and spice blends for sweet and savoury cooking. All are Australian Certified Organic. I created them to help my clients make beautiful food without the use of processed ingredients and additives found in pre-made condiments, sauces, pastes and stocks. With the exception of the All Things Nice Blend, they all come in their coarse state so either use them whole or grind them in a mortar and pestle.

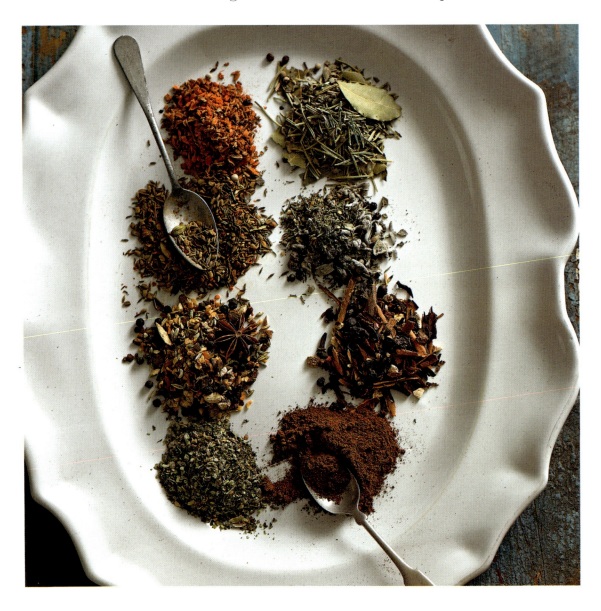

All Things Nice
Vanilla bean, allspice, cinnamon and nutmeg powders. A fragrant blend of sweet spices to sprinkle onto custard, ice-cream or yoghurt or add to smoothies. Also adds a lovely flavour to cakes, biscuits or French toast.

Fragrant Fruit
Elderberries, hawthorn berries, rosehips, nutmeg powder, cinnamon powder, cloves buds, hibiscus flowers and orange peel. A rich, fragrant blend of fruit and spices that is perfect for poaching fruit, making mulled wine or a rich syrup for cakes, porridge, yoghurt or custard.

Grecian
Rosemary leaves, bay leaves, black and white peppercorns and garlic granules. A Greek-inspired blend for roast vegetables, fish and meat, particularly roast lamb. Make a delicious salad dressing when combined with olive oil and fresh lemon juice.

Indian
Cumin seeds, turmeric powder, cardamom pods, fennel seeds, fenugreek, black peppercorns, cinnamon chips, chilli flakes and garlic granules. This Indian-inspired blend is perfect for slow-cooked curries and braises, allowing the spices time to infuse. Add a cooling yoghurt.

Mexican
Paprika powder, chilli flakes, cumin seeds, oregano leaves, black peppercorns and garlic granules. This fiery Mexican inspired blend is delicious on meat and vegetables. Adds an authentic Mexican flavour to salsa or guacamole.

Oriental
Star anise, fennel seeds, cloves, black peppercorns, cinnamon chips and garlic granules. This aromatic, Asian-inspired blend is perfect on chicken, duck and orange slices or pork and apple. It creates a sweet, crispy skin.

Provincial
Sage leaves, thyme leaves, black and white peppercorns and garlic granules. Try on scrambled eggs, baked vegetables or with chicken. Add to olive oil and lemon juice for a salad dressing or mix with yoghurt to make a sauce for poached salmon.

Sunday Roast
Celtic sea salt, rosemary leaves, thyme leaves, sage leaves, bay leaves, garlic granules and cracked black peppercorn. Rub onto beef, lamb, pork, poultry, fish and vegetables for succulent traditional roasts.

Tuscan
Basil leaves, marjoram leaves, oregano leaves, black peppercorns and garlic granules. A traditional Italian-inspired blend for sauteed or roast meats, poultry or fish. Perfect in tomato-based dishes.

Resources

A select list of reading material if you are interested in following up any of the issues raised in this book.

General

Fallon, S. *Nourishing traditions*, New Trends Publishing Inc, Washington D.C. 2001, mercola.com

Aquaculture

Duffy, C. and Bryan, S. 'Salmon: Clean, green super-food or battery hens of the sea?', abc.net.au

Fisheries and Aquaculture Department, 'The production of fish meal and oil', fao.org/docrep

Breast milk substitute (homemade)

westonaprice.org/childrens-health/recipes-for-homemade-baby-formula

Carcinogens in non-stick cookware

Steenland K., Woskie S., 'Cohort mortality study of workers exposed to perfluorooctonoic acid', ncbi.nlm.nih.gov/pubmed

Chemicals in food

Biopharmaceutics & Drug Disposition, vol. 16, 351–380 (1995).

Erisman, J. W.; Sutton, M.A.; Galloway, J.; Klimont Z.; Winiwarter W. 'How a century of ammonia synthesis changed the world'. *Nature Geoscience* 1 (10): 636.

The Journal of the American Nutraceutical Association, vol. 5, no. 3 Summer 2002.

Chocolate

'Cocoa Market Update', World Cocoa Foundation, May 2010.

Choline

Boynton, E., 'Nutrients in Eggs and Meat May Influence Gene Expression from Infancy to Adulthood', urmc.rochester.edu

Vishnudutt Purohit, Manal F. Abdelmalek, Shirish Barve, Norlin J. Benevenga, Charles H. Halsted, Neil Kaplowitz, Kusum K. Kharbanda, Qi-Ying Liu, Shelly C. Lu, Craig J. McClain, Christine Swanson, and Samir Zakhari, 'Role of S-adenosylmethionine, folate, and betaine in the treatment of alcoholic liver disease', ajcn.nutrition.org

Dangers of burnt food

Larsson, B. K.; Sahlberg, G.P.; Eriksson, A.T.; Busk, L.A. (1983). 'Polycyclic aromatic hydrocarbons in grilled food.' *Journal of Agricultural and Food Chemistry*. 31 (4): 867–873.

Polycyclic Aromatic Hydrocarbons – Occurrence in foods, dietary exposure and health effects. European Commission, Scientific Committee on Food. December 4, 2002.

Dangers of microwaves

Song K., Milner J.A., 'The influence of heating on the anticancer properties of garlic', ncbi.nlm.nih.gov/pubmed

F. Vallejo, F.A. Tomás-Barberán, C. García-Viguera, 'Phenolic compound contents in edible parts of broccoli inflorescences after domestic cooking', onlinelibrary.wiley.com

Powerwatch, 'Microwave Oven and Microwave Cooking Overview' powerwatch.org.uk

Fats

westonaprice.org/know-your-fats/know-your-fats-introduction

Food acids

MBM Food Additives Guide, mbm.net.au/health/guide.htm

Fructose

Hanover, L.M.; White, J.S. 'Manufacturing, composition, and application of fructose', *Journal of Clinical Nutrition* 58: 724s–732, Oregon State University (1993).

Genetics

Frances A. Champagne, Ian C. G. Weaver, Josie Diorio, Sergiy Dymov, Moshe Szyf and Michael J. Meaney, 'Maternal Care Associated with Methylation of the Estrogen Receptor-α1b Promoter and

Estrogen Receptor-α Expression in the Medial Preoptic Area of Female Offspring', endo.endojournals.org

Bruce S. McEwen and Peter J. Gianaros, 'Central role of the brain in stress and adaptation: Links to socioeconomic status, health, and disease,' ncbi.nlm.nih.gov

Christian Caldji, Ian C. Hellstrom, Tie-Yuan Zhang, Josie Diorio, Michael J. Meaney, 'Environmental regulation of the neural epigenome', sciencedirect.com

Frances A. Champagne, James P. Curley, 'How social experiences influence the brain', sciencedirect.com

Heirloom seeds

diggers.com.au

edenseeds.com.au

Herbal remedies and supplements

ausflowers.com.au

bachflower.com

Bone, K. *The Ultimate Herbal Compendium*, Phytotherapy Press, 2007

Malini, T.; Arunakaran, J.; Aruldhas, M.M.; Govindarajulu, P.; 'Effects of piperine on the lipid composition and enzymes of the pyruvate-malate cycle in the testis of the rat in vivo'. *Biochemistry and Molecular Biology Education* Int 1999; 47(3): 537-45

martinandpleasance.com/brands/schuessler-tissue-salts/

Hexane toxicity

The Cornucopia Institute, *Soy Report and Scorecard*, cornucopia.org

Irradiated food

foodandwaterwatch.org/food/irradiation/irradiation-facts

foodirradiationwatch.org/fact-sheets

Meat

L. Wyness, E. Weichselbaum, A. O'Connor, E. B. Williams, 'Red meat in the diet: an update', onlinelibrary.wiley.com

Nitrates in bacon

chriskresser.com/the-nitrate-and-nitrite-myth-another-reason-not-to-fear-bacon

Nuts

chriskresser.com/another-reason-you-shouldnt-go-nuts-on-nuts

Paleolithic diet

Chriskresser.com

Crane, E. *The Archaeology of Beekeeping*, Cornell University Press (1983)

primalbody-primalmind.com

'Stone Age Had Beer', *Popular Science Magazine* (1931).

Yerkes, R. M. *The Great Apes*. New Haven, Yale University Press, 1929.

Raw milk

Braun-Fahrländer, C., Von Mutius, E. 'Can farm milk consumption prevent allergic diseases?', *Clinical and Experimental Allergy*, Volume 41, Issue 1, 29–35 (January 2011).

Seasonal eating

Haas, E.M. *Staying healthy with the seasons*, Celestial Arts, New York, 2003.

Thickeners

MBM, *Food Additives Guide*, mbm.net.au

Stress

Schocker, L., 'This is your body on stress', huffingtonpost.com

Salt

Breslin, P. A. S.; Beauchamp, G. K. 'Salt enhances flavour by suppressing bitterness', *Nature*, Volume 387, Issue 6633, 563, 1997.

Zinc

Tapiero, H., Tew K.D., 'Trace elements in human physiology and pathology: zinc and metallothioneins', www.ncbi.nlm.nih.gov/pubmed

General index

A
acid/alkaline diet 8
'activated' nuts and seeds 43
agar-agar 204
alcohol 52, 57
allergen-free diet 8
almond meal 213
antibiotics 25
anticaking agents 25
antifoaming agents 25
antinutrients 35
antioxidants 71
apple cider vinegar 93
apricots 28
artichokes 103
artificial sweeteners 53
ascorbic acid 26
aspartame 26

B
baking 29, 34
barbecuing 29
beta-carotene 9
biodynamic farming 19
biotin 81
bisphenol A 31
bitters 52
bleaches 25
braising 32
bran 46
bread improvers 45
breakfast cereals 45
buckwheat 46
butter 58

C
caffeine 57
calcium 74
canned goods 31
canola oil (rapeseed) 23
carbohydrates 4
carotenoid antioxidants 111
casseroles 32, 34
chemical extraction 31
chemical ingredients 25
chemical-free foods 20
chicken
   buying 38, 58
children, food for 5
cholesterol-lowering diets 8
choline 74
citric acid 26
cleansing 4, 66–9
coconut oil 42, 82
cod liver oil 42
coeliac disease 46
coffee 52
   substitutes 46
condiments 49
constipation 46
convenience foods 4, 11
cooking techniques to avoid 29–32
corn 11
corn oil 23
crackers, store-bought 45–6

D
dairy foods 57
   buying 58
   lactose intolerance 22, 40
   raw 34
deli meats 38–9, 58
detox process 59
diets, types of 7–8
digestive system 59
dioxins 20
dried fruit 28, 38
dried herbs and spices 235–6
   blends 239
drinks 52–3
   coffee 46, 52
   fizzy 53
   soft drinks 53
   sports drinks 53
   tea 53
   water 52

E
eating disorders 7
eggs 11
   buying 58
   health benefits 84
   raw 34, 81
electrolytes 49
emulsifiers 25
endotoxins 108
extra virgin oil 42

F
factory farming 12
farmers' markets 14
fats, buying 58
fermenting 34–5
   fermented drinks 93
fibre 46
fish
   farmed salmon 12–13
   omega 3 and 6 levels 12
   raw 34
   sustainable 12, 13, 146
fish oil 12, 42
fizzy drinks 53
flaxseed oil 42
flour, white 23, 25
food acids 26
food allergy 8
food choices 5, 14
food colours 26
food enhancers 26
food flavourings 26
food intolerance 8
food irradiation 19
food philosophies (top 10) 4–5
Food Standards Australia and New Zealand 39
fossil fuels 14
free radicals 71
fructose malabsorption 22
fruit 57
   choosing 37, 58
   frozen 37
frying 29

G
genetically modified foods 4, 19
gluten intolerance 46
goat's milk 30
goitrogens 34, 35
grains 45, 58
   forms 43
   phytic acids 43
   processed 57
   sprouting 35
grapefruit juice 93
grapeseed oil 23
grazing 59
green vegetables 9
Greenpeace 39
grilling 29
gubinge powder 208
gut flora 4

H
health food diet 7
'health foods' 45–6
healthy eating, basic steps 9
heavy metals 2
heirloom seeds 13
herbal tea 53, 59, 65, 93
   blends 231
   a perfect cup 231
herbs
   A–Z of 234–7
   blends 238–9
   fresh 43, 232
high fructose corn syrup 22
homogenisation 30
honey 50
hormone-free foods 20
humectanting agents 25
hunter-gatherers 55
hydrogen cyanide 35
hydrogenation 30

I
immune system 75

J
juices 52–3, 93
juicing diets 9

L
lamb 58
lactase 40
lactose intolerance 22, 40
lectins 35
legumes, buying 58
liquorice 46
'locavore' 14
long-life products 30

M
magnesium 75
Maillard reaction 30, 29
malnutrition 2
Marine Conservation 13, 148
meal planning 56
meal 'replacements' 8, 27
meat
   fat in 38
   from grass-fed animals 12, 14, 19
   'organic' 16, 19
   raw 34
   red or white 38
   well-done, charred 29
medications, over-the-counter 57
meditation 68
menu plan (28-day) 59–63
microwaving 31–2
milk
   goats' milk 30, 40
   long-life 40
   lactose-free 40
   lactose intolerance 22, 40
   homogenised 30
   unhomogenised 30
milk solids 22
minerals 2
MSG 57
muesli
   Bircher-style 45
muesli bars, store-bought 45–6

N
'natural' ingredients 22–5
neotame 26
non-stick cookware 29
nutritional deficiencies 2
nutritional density 2, 4
nuts 58
   'activated' 43

iodine 35, 49, 75
iron 75
irradiation-free foods 19

butters 43
raw 43
sprouting 35

O
oils and fats 43, 58
 cold pressed 31, 42
 plant fats 40
 saturated 40, 42
 vegetable 31
omega 3 fatty acids 42
omega 6 fatty acids 8
organic farming 4, 16–19
oxalates 34, 35

P
pan-frying 32
pasteurised products 30
peanut oil 23
pepper 232, 236
periodic eating 13–14
permaculture 19
pesticides 1, 20
pH level 4, 8
phytates 2
phytic acid 35, 45, 50
pickles 38
plant fats 42
preservatives 26
processed food 2
 grains 57
 omega 6 fatty acids 8
 and shelf life 20
 stocktake of 56
protein bars 27
protein powders 27

pseudocereals 43, 46, 89

R
raw food 4, 34
 diet 9–10
rice cakes 45

S
saccharin 26
salt 49, 232
sashimi 136
saturated fats 159
sausages 58
sauteing 32
seafood
 buying 39, 58
 pre-cooked, frozen 39
 sashimi 136
 sustainable 13, 39
seasonal affective disorder 69
seasonal eating 14, 59, 66, 67, 68
seasonings 58, 232
 see also spices
seaweed 49, 58, 124
seeds
 'activated' 43
 buying 43
 preparing 213
 sprouting 35
selenium 75
sesame oil 23
shopping list 58
simmering 32
slow-roasting 34
snacks 56
soft drinks 53

soup 32
sourdough bread 45
soy 23, 49
spices 43, 58
 A–Z of 234–7
 blends 238–9
 dried 235–6
 see also dried herbs and spices
sports drinks 53
spreads and pastes 58
sprouting 35
 sprouted bread 45
starch 23
steaming 32
sterilising jars 122
stevia 26, 50, 58, 237
stewing 32
stir-fries 29
sucralose 26
sugar, eliminating 57
'sugar-free' products 22
sunflower oil 23
'super foods' 57
supplements 5, 7, 57
sustainable wholefood, choosing 28, 37, 38–9, 40, 42
sweeteners 11, 26, 50, 58

T
table salt 23
table sugar 23
tea 53
 teabags 53
thickeners 26–7, 46
transfats 30
trypsin inhibitors 35

28-day menu plan 59–63

U
ultraheating (UHT) 30
umami 160
unprocessed food 4, 20

V
vegetable oils 23
 see also plant fats
vegetables
 choosing 58
 frozen 37
 seasonal eating 66–9
vinegar 58
 apple cider vinegar 93
vitamins 71–4, 159

W
water 52
water filters 53
weight-loss diets 7–8
wholefoods, fresh 4
wholefood diet 4
wine 52
wok-fries 29

Y
yeast 22, 57
yoghurt 58, 82

Z
zinc 75

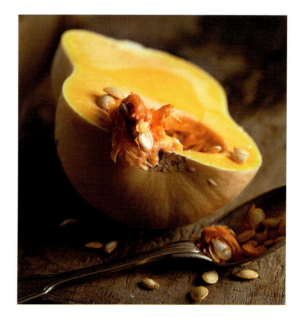

Recipe index

A

Aioli 224
almond cakes
   Cinnamon apple almond cake 186
   Spiced apple coconut cake 189
   Vanilla banana coconut cake 189
   Vanilla orange almond cake 186
   Vanilla pear almond cake 186
amaranth 46
   Moroccan spice quinoa and amaranth 121
Aphrodite's delight (yoghurt) 218
apple
   Apple and blueberry crumble 195
   Apple, fennel and celery salad 115
   Cinnamon apple almond cake 186
   Roast pork belly with apple, cabbage and fennel 169
   Spiced apple coconut cake 189
asparagus 103
avocado
   Velvety lime avocado dip 99

B

Baked eggs 85
   Baked eggs with tomato and haloumi 153
Baked fennel sausages with eggplants and tomato 151
Baked fish with fennel, onion and parsley 146
bananas
   Vanilla banana coconut cake 189
beef
   Beef carpaccio with radish and celery 139
   Beef short ribs with Sunday Roast Blend 176
   Mexican fajita lettuce wraps 142
   searing 167
   Slow-cooked spicy beef coconut pumpkin curry 172
   Steak tartare 135
beetroot
   Beet kvass 53, 223
   Beet leaves with walnuts 106
   Fresh beetroot, egg and rocket salad 104
berries
   Apple and blueberry crumble 195
biscuits 45
   Chocolate and pear biscuit 198
   Parmesan biscuits 196
   Pear and coconut slice 198
Blackened eggplant dip 99
bok choy (Chinese broccoli) 103
breakfast beverages 93
broccoli 103
brussels sprouts 103

C

cabbage
   Fermented cabbage, carrots and caraway seeds 221
   Roast pork belly with apple, cabbage and fennel 169
   steamed 103
cakes
   Chocolate cloud cake 190
   Cinnamon apple almond cake 186
   Zucchini and carrot cake with lemon vanilla cream-cheese icing 192
   see also almond cakes
carrots
   Classic French grated carrots 108
   Fermented cabbage, carrots and caraway seeds 221
   Orange butter carrots 108
   raw 108
   Zucchini and carrot cake with lemon vanilla cream-cheese icing 192
cauliflower
   Smooth cauliflower mash 111
celery
   Apple, fennel and celery salad 115
   Beef carpaccio with radish and celery 139
   Leek and celery soup 131
chard 103
cheese 40, 58
   Baked eggs with tomato and haloumi 153
   Parmesan biscuits 196
   see also cream cheese
chicken
   Chicken, egg and lemon soup 127
   giblets 178
   gravy 178
   Indian spiced chicken with spinach 156
   Roast chicken 178
   Salt and pepper chilli chicken with lime 154
   Spicy lemon butter chicken legs 154
   stuffing 178
   thigh fillets 154
Chicken liver pate 228
chilli 235
   Salt and pepper chilli chicken with lime 154
Chinese broccoli, steamed 103
chocolate 50, 58
   Chocolate cloud cake 190
   Chocolate coconut macaroons 184
   Chocolate ice-cream 201
   Chocolate mousse 201
   Chocolate and pear biscuit 198
   fruit dipped in 199
   Homemade 'chocolate' 199
Cinnamon apple almond cake 186
Clear broth 124
coconut
   Chocolate coconut macaroons 184
   Coconut cream (drink) 199
   Coconut cream (ice-cream) 199
   Coconut crumble 195
   Coconut macaroons 184
   Coconut oil and lime juice dressing 117
   Fragrant coconut soup with seafood 129
   Orange coconut macaroons 184
   Pear and coconut slice 198
   Slow-cooked spicy beef coconut pumpkin curry 172
   Spiced apple coconut cake 189
   Vanilla banana coconut cake 189
cream cheese
   Lemon vanilla cream-cheese icing 192
crumble
   Apple and blueberry crumble 195
   Coconut crumble 195
cucumber
   Cucumber, ruby grapefruit and witlof salad 115
   Minty cucumber yoghurt dip 99
   Roast duck, cucumber, orange and pomegranate salad 162
   Tomato with fresh curd and cucumber ribbons 115
cultured vegetables
   Beet kvass 53, 223
   Fermented cabbage, carrots and caraway seeds 221
   Kefir yoghurt drink 223
   Pickled ginger 222
curd
   Tomato with fresh curd and cucumber ribbons 115
   see also fresh curds and whey
curry
   Slow-cooked spicy beef coconut pumpkin curry 172

D

dips
   Blackened eggplant dip 99
   Green tahini dip 99
   Minty cucumber yoghurt dip 99
   Velvety lime avocado dip 99
dressings, quick 117
   Coconut oil and lime juice dressing 117
   Garlic, lemon and tahini dressing 117
   Olive oil and lemon juice dressing 117
   Orange, mustard and yoghurt dressing 117
drinks
   Beet kvass 223
   Coconut cream 199
   fermented 93
   Kefir yoghurt drink 223
   Smoothies 81, 215
duck 58
   Duck and grapefruit lettuce wraps 161
   Oriental duck soup 160
   Roast duck 159
   Roast duck, cucumber, orange and pomegranate salad 162
duck fat 159

E

eggplant
    Baked fennel sausages with eggplants and tomato 151
    Blackened eggplant dip 99
eggs
    Baked eggs 85
    Baked eggs with tomato and haloumi 153
    Chicken, egg and lemon soup 127
    Fresh beetroot, egg and rocket salad 104
    Hard-boiled eggs 85
    Lightly pan-fried eggs 85
    Omelette or scrambled eggs 85
    Poached eggs 85
    Soft-boiled eggs 85
Elderflower and kiwi popsicles 208

F

fennel
    Apple, fennel and celery salad 115
    Baked fennel sausages with eggplants and tomato 151
    Baked fish with fennel, onion and parsley 146
    Roast pork belly with apple, cabbage and fennel 169
    seeds 235
Fermented cabbage, carrots and caraway seeds 221
fish
    Baked fish with fennel, onion and parsley 146
    cooking times 145
    Fish fillets with sage and butter 145
    Raw marinated sardines with zesty tomato 150
    Tuna fillet in a jar 122
Fragrant coconut soup with seafood 129
Fragrant poached fruit 199
Fresh beetroot, egg and rocket salad 104
fresh curds and whey 216
Fresh tomato and basil soup 131
frittata
    Lemon, capsicum and zucchini frittata 134
fruit
    dipped in chocolate 199
    Fragrant fruit yoghurt 82
    Fragrant poached fruit 199
    Fruit jelly 204

G

garlic
    Aioli 224
    Garlic, lemon and tahini dressing 117
    granules 236
    Lentil, lemon and garlic soup 132
gelatin 202, 215
ginger 236
    Pickled ginger 222
    Pumpkin and ginger soup 131
Gluten-free porridge 89
grapefruit
    Cucumber, ruby grapefruit and witlof salad 115
    Duck and grapefruit lettuce wraps 161

Green tahini dip 99
green vegetables
    Leafy greens and herb salad 115
    Steamed greens 103

H

herbs
    Fresh tomato and basil soup 131
    Herb mayonnaise 224
    Leafy greens and herb salad 115
    Tabouli sans grain 118

I

ice-cream
    Chocolate ice-cream 201
    Coconut cream 199
icing
    Lemon vanilla cream-cheese icing 192

J

jelly
    Fruit jelly 204
    Old-fashioned gummy jellies 205
    Sweet gummy jellies 205
    Sweet and sour gummy jellies 205
    Real jelly 202
    Tea jelly 204
    with fruit 205

K

kale 103
Kefir yoghurt drink 223
kiwi fruit
    Elderflower and kiwi popsicles 208

L

lamb
    Marinated lamb chops 170
    Pan-fried lamb cutlets 168
    Roast leg of lamb 181
    Slow-cooked Tuscan lamb shanks 175
Leafy greens and herb salad 115
Leek and celery soup 131
leftovers
    Leftover roast salad 100
    Warm leftovers 100
lemons
    Chicken, egg and lemon soup 127
    Garlic, lemon and tahini dressing 117
    juice 93
    Lemon, capsicum and zucchini frittata 134
    Lemon vanilla cream-cheese icing 192
    Lentil, lemon and garlic soup 132
    Olive oil and lemon juice dressing 117
Lentil, lemon and garlic soup 132
lettuce
    Duck and grapefruit lettuce wraps 161
    Mexican fajita lettuce wraps 142
    Pan-fried radicchio or baby cos with garlic lemon dressing 106
Lightly pan-fried eggs 85
lime
    Coconut oil and lime juice dressing 117
    juice 93
    Salt and pepper chilli chicken with lime 154

Velvety lime avocado dip 99

M

macaroons
    Chocolate coconut macaroons 184
    Orange coconut macaroons 184
Marinated lamb chops 170
mash
    Smooth cauliflower mash 111
    Sweet potato mash with cinnamon 111
Mayonnaise 224
    Aioli 224
    Herb 224
meatballs
    Sweet onion meatballs 164
Mexican fajita lettuce wraps 142
Minty cucumber yoghurt dip 99
Moroccan spice quinoa and amaranth 121
mousse
    Chocolate mousse 201
muesli
    Pear and vanilla bircher 90
    Traditional 90
mustard
    Dijon 224
    Orange, mustard and yoghurt dressing 117

N

nuts
    Orange, rosewater and pistachio with vanilla yoghurt 206
    see also almonds; walnuts

O

omelettes
    Omelette or scrambled eggs 85
    Sweet berry omelette 85
onions
    Baked fish with fennel, onion and parsley 146
    Sweet onion meatballs 164
oranges
    Orange butter carrots 108
    Orange coconut macaroons 184
    Orange, mustard and yoghurt dressing 117
    Orange, rosewater and pistachio with vanilla yoghurt 206
    Roast duck, cucumber, orange and pomegranate salad 162
    Vanilla orange almond cake 186
Osso buco 175

P

Panna cotta 204
Parmesan biscuits 196
parsley
    Tabouli sans grain 118
pears
    Chocolate and pear biscuit 198
    Pear and coconut slice 198
    Pear and vanilla bircher 90
    Vanilla pear almond cake 186
Pickled ginger 222
popsicles
    Elderflower and kiwi popsicles 208

fruity variations 208
pork 58
    Roast pork belly with apple, cabbage and fennel 169
porridge
    Gluten-free porridge 89
prawns
    Pan-fried spice prawns with cherry tomatoes 148
    Prawn and scallop ceviche 136
Provincial roast vegetable salad 112
pumpkin
    Pumpkin and ginger soup 131
    Slow-cooked spicy beef coconut pumpkin curry 172

Q
quinoa 46
    Moroccan spice quinoa and amaranth 121

R
radicchio
    Pan-fried radicchio or baby cos with garlic lemon dressing 106
radish
    Beef carpaccio with radish and celery 139
Raw marinated sardines with zesty tomato 150
roasts
    Leftover roast salad 100
    Roast chicken 178
    Roast duck 159
    Roast duck, cucumber, orange and pomegranate salad 162
    Roast leg of lamb 181
    Roast pork belly with apple, cabbage and fennel 169
rocket
    Fresh beetroot, egg and rocket salad 104

S
salads
    Apple, fennel and celery salad 115
    Cucumber, ruby grapefruit and witlof salad 115
    Fresh beetroot, egg and rocket salad 104
    Leafy greens and herb salad 115
    Leftover roast salad 100
    Provincial roast vegetable salad 112
    Roast duck, cucumber, orange and pomegranate salad 162
    Tomato with fresh curd and cucumber ribbons 115
Salt and pepper chilli chicken with lime 154

sausages
    Baked fennel sausages with eggplants and tomato 151
seafood
    Fragrant coconut soup with seafood 129
    see also prawns
silverbeet 103
Slow-cooked spicy beef coconut pumpkin curry 172
Slow-cooked Tuscan lamb shanks 175
Smooth cauliflower mash 111
Smoothies 81, 215
soup
    broths 93
    Chicken, egg and lemon soup 127
    Clear broth 124
    Fragrant coconut soup with seafood 129
    Fresh tomato and basil soup 131
    garnishes 131
    Leek and celery soup 131
    Lentil, lemon and garlic soup 132
    Oriental duck soup 160
    Pumpkin and ginger soup 131
    Vegetable soup 131
spices
    Indian spiced chicken with spinach 156
    Moroccan spice quinoa and amaranth 121
    Pan-fried spice prawns with cherry tomatoes 148
    Spice Yoghurt 82
    Spiced apple coconut cake 189
    Spicy lemon butter chicken legs 154
spinach
    Indian spiced chicken with spinach 156
    steamed 103
sprouts 213
steak 167
    Steak tartare 135
Steamed greens 103
stock 100
    making your own 214–15
Sweet and sour gummy jellies 205
Sweet gummy jellies 205
Sweet onion meatballs 164
Sweet potato mash with cinnamon 111

T
Tabouli sans grain 118
tahini
    Garlic, lemon and tahini dressing 117
    Green tahini dip 99
Tea jelly 204
tomatoes
    Baked eggs with tomato and haloumi 153

Fresh tomato and basil soup 131
Pan-fried spice prawns with cherry tomatoes 148
Raw marinated sardines with zesty tomato 150
Tabouli sans grain 118
Tomato with fresh curd and cucumber ribbons 115
Tomato sauce 227
Tropical yoghurt 82
Tuna fillet in a jar 122

V
Vanilla banana coconut cake 189
Vanilla orange almond cake 186
Vanilla pear almond cake 186
Vanilla yoghurt 206
veal
    Osso buco 175
vegetables
    Provincial roast vegetable salad 112
    Vegetable soup 131
    see also cultured vegetables; green vegetables; mash, specific vegetables
Velvety lime avocado dip 99

W
witlof
    Cucumber, ruby grapefruit and witlof salad 115
wraps
    Duck and grapefruit lettuce wraps 161
    Mexican fajita lettuce wraps 142

Y
yoghurt
    Aphrodite's delight 218
    Fragrant fruit yoghurt 82
    Homemade Greek yoghurt 218
    Kefir yoghurt drink 222
    Minty cucumber yoghurt dip 99
    Orange, mustard and yoghurt dressing 117
    Orange, rosewater and pistachio with vanilla yoghurt 206
    Tropical yoghurt 82
    Spice yoghurt 82
    Vanilla yoghurt 206

Z
zucchini 103
    Lemon, capsicum and zucchini frittata 134
    Zucchini and carrot cake with lemon vanilla cream-cheese icing 192

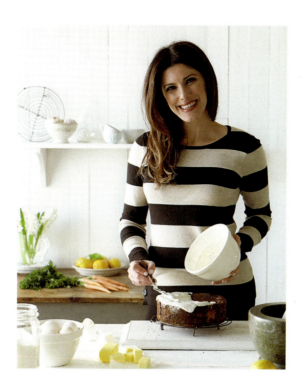

Acknowledgements

Thank you for your wisdom, inspiration, support,
love and food for my heart, mind and tummy:

Paavo Airola, Weston A. Price, Sally Fallon, Paul Chek, John McGrath,
Martin Boetz, Julie Gibbs, Victoria Alexander, Alice Waters, Penelope Sach,
Alana Mann, Natalie Lascelles and Kennedy Gandhi.

Penguin dream team: Rachel, Jocelyn, Katrina, Chris, Daniel, Vanessa
and everyone else involved in the creation of my beautiful book.

My Ovvio girls: Catie, Ashley, Linda, Junko.

My mum and dad, Andrew and Irene and my brother Eric.

My partner, Paul Cheika.

My grandparents, my aunties and my big family.

My furry kids, Casper and Maya.

LANTERN

UK | USA | Canada | Ireland | Australia
India | New Zealand | South Africa | China

Penguin Books is part of the Penguin Random House group of companies whose addresses
can be found at global.penguinrandomhouse.com.

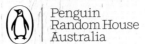

First published by Penguin Group (Australia), 2014

3 5 7 9 10 8 6 4 2

Text copyright   Anthia Koullouros 2014

The moral right of the author has been asserted.

All rights reserved. Without limiting the rights under copyright reserved above, no part of this
publication may be reproduced, stored in or introduced into a retrieval system, or
transmitted, in any form or by any means (electronic, mechanical, photocopying, recording or
otherwise), without the prior written permission of both the copyright owner and the above publisher of this book.

Cover and text design by Daniel New © Penguin Group (Australia)
Cover and author photographs © Chris Chen
Photography by Chris L. Jones except for pages 6, 21, 64, 70, 78, 91, 94, 101, 105, 107, 109,
110, 119, 120, 133, 140, 152, 174, 177, 182, 191, 193, 197, 203, 207, 209, 210, 219, 226, 230, 240
© Chris Chen, pages 12, 16, 23, 29 by iStock and page 26 by Shutterstock.
Typeset in Baskerville by Post Pre-Press, Brisbane
Colour reproduction by Splitting Image Colour Studio, Clayton, Victoria
Printed and bound in China by Everbest Printing Co Ltd.

National Library of Australia
Cataloguing-in-Publication data:

Koullouros, Anthia, author.

I am food/Anthia Koullouros.

ISBN 9781921383953 (paperback)

Includes bibliographical references and index

Food habits.
Natural foods.
Nutrition.
Food in popular culture.
641.3

penguin.com.au/lantern